T0355562

The Terry Lectures

A Way of Life

Volumes in the Terry Lectures Series Available from
Yale University Press

For a full list of titles in print in the Terry Lectures Series, visit
yalebooks.com or yaleup.co.uk.

A WAY OF LIFE

THINGS, THOUGHT, AND
ACTION IN CHINESE MEDICINE

JUDITH FARQUHAR

Yale

UNIVERSITY PRESS

New Haven and London

Published with assistance from the Louis Stern Memorial Fund.

Yale University Press books may be purchased in quantity for
educational, business, or promotional use. For information, please e-mail
sales.press@yale.edu (U.S. office) or sales@yaleup.co.uk (U.K. office).

Set in Adobe Garamond type by Newgen North America.
Printed in the United States of America.

Library of Congress Control Number: 2019944796
ISBN 978-0-300-23723-8 (hardcover : alk. paper)

A catalogue record for this book is available from the British Library.

This paper meets the requirements of ANSI/NISO Z39.48-1992
(Permanence of Paper).

10 9 8 7 6 5 4 3 2 1

The Dwight Harrington Terry Foundation Lectures on Religion in the Light of Science and Philosophy

The deed of gift declares that "the object of this foundation is not the promotion of scientific investigation and discovery, but rather the assimilation and interpretation of that which has been or shall be hereafter discovered, and its application to human welfare, especially by the building of the truths of science and philosophy into the structure of a broadened and purified religion. The founder believes that such a religion will greatly stimulate intelligent effort for the improvement of human conditions and the advancement of the race in strength and excellence of character. To this end it is desired that a series of lectures be given by men eminent in their respective departments, on ethics, the history of civilization and religion, biblical research, all sciences and branches of knowledge which have an important bearing on the subject, all the great laws of nature, especially of evolution . . . also such interpretations of literature and sociology as are in accord with the spirit of this foundation, to the end that the Christian spirit may be nurtured in the fullest light of the world's knowledge and that mankind may be helped to attain its highest possible welfare and happiness upon this earth." The present work constitutes the latest volume published on this foundation.

本立而道生

If the root is sound, the Way can come to life.

Lu Guangxin, *The Way of Chinese Medicine*, 5

Contents

Acknowledgments

I wish to express special thanks to Dale Martin for nominating me to deliver the Terry Lectures at Yale in the fall of 2017. We had shared interests in reading obscure sources for "the body" many years before that, and it has been wonderful to renew our exchanges on this and related subjects in New Haven and since then. Dale understands, better than almost anyone, the frustrations and joys of thinking differently by way of engagement with a literature remote from the modern West. His support for my explorations in Chinese medicine has been crucial in the writing of this book.

Also at Yale in 2017, the members of the Terry Lectures Committee were kind hosts and interesting interlocutors. During my stay in New Haven I learned much that was of use for this project from David Luesink, Valerie Hansen, James van Pelt, Mary Evelyn Tucker, Deborah Davis, Helen Siu, and an unbelievably generous Hazel Carby. Jean Thomson Black of Yale University Press provided much-appreciated support throughout the lectures and the preparation of this book.

In some respects these lectures were a humble translation project, as I have relied heavily on the writing of Chinese scholars and doctors in my efforts to characterize "things, thought, and action" in Chinese medicine. Some of the many experts whose writing has been germinal in my own work are cited in this volume. I hope readers will begin to see, through them, how rich the literature of Chinese medicine is when viewed by way of this little window of philosophy in translation.

In Beijing, Lili Lai continues to push me toward writing and publishing better explanations of Chinese medicine. Liu Cheng constantly surprises me with his outside-the-box insights about medicine and health. Colin Garon, who first became my comrade in Chinese medicine in Chicago, is still feeding me observations and interpretations from his clinical and classroom perches in Beijing. Zhang Dong of the China Academy of Chinese Medical Sciences, author of appendix 2, is a new inspiration in my philosophical life. Thank you, all.

I have met periodically in recent years with the Translating Vitalities Collective, benefiting much from the creative collaborations that have joined us since 2012. I hope my TV comrades will see *A Way of Life* as a valid contribution to our ongoing concert, along with the sillier experiment "Bee-Coming Unfolded" with Larisa Jasarevic and the work of the Space Crafters Volker Scheid, Clare Twomey, Suzanne Cochrane, and Vincent Duclos that appeared in *Somatosphere* (www.translatingvitalities.com).

In Chicago, James Hevia read the whole book as it emerged, keeping me going with his rapid and helpful edits. Heangjin Park combined brilliant manuscript preparation services with enjoyable speculative conversations. And Anne Ch'ien kept reminding me that working closely with Chinese sources is eternally worth it. Though these lectures could have been prepared only by me, they are quietly indebted to all this precious companionship.

A Way of Life

Science, Civilization, and Practice in and beyond Chinese Medicine

There is, it must be confessed, a curious fascination in hearing
deep things talked about, even tho neither we nor the disputants
understand them. We get the problematic thrill, we feel the presence of the vastness.

William James, *Pragmatism*

The Dwight H. Terry Lectures at Yale, which since 1923 have
been asking us to think science and religion together, offer a precious opportunity to hear deep things talked about. This book is expanded from the 2017 Terry Lectures in which I spoke about things,
thought, and action in and beyond Chinese medicine. In three lectures, I presented some Chinese approaches to these fundamental
concerns as posing questions important not only in the worlds of
traditional medicine but also to human experience in general.

I have reasons for this way of exploring things, thought, and action: I can clearly remember the moment in 1982 when I first started
to read about Chinese medicine in Chinese. Sitting in a hot dormi-
tory room at the Guangzhou College of Traditional Chinese Medicine, facing a stack of new textbooks brought to me by an advisor,
I was startled and delighted to realize that I had suddenly gained

access—simply by opening some books and reading—to a reality, a rationality, and a form of ethical action that had previously been almost entirely unknown to me.

Much of my academic career since then has been devoted to unspooling and reliving the joy I felt that evening as I began to read, and much of my writing has aimed to fulfill the deep and grateful obligation I feel to my teachers in that college. They and those textbooks—some of which were authored by those same teachers—opened a new world and a new way of thinking to me.[1] In this book, then, I continue my efforts to better understand, and translate for all manner of "disputants," the logic and practice of Chinese medicine. Though I have found this material to be quite clear when it is read in modern textbook Chinese, much of what I know about the field is rather technical and difficult to understand in English. So be warned! Not being a doctor, or a healer of any kind, I think of myself as an impassioned translator of lived worlds. I hope my translations between languages and worlds can speak to readers who are curious about many things, some of them deep. Perhaps I can persuade all who might be fascinated by "hearing deep things talked about" that an ancient and ever-changing Asian language, unfamiliar forms of embodiment, and lively arenas of contemporary practice can be made more accessible to our imaginations by anthropological research on "traditional" medicine in China. In a sense, this set of lectures and this book are an effort to re-invoke, for myself and I hope for my readers, the "problematic thrill" of thinking in fresh ways about hard-to-understand things. Perhaps Chinese medicine, alongside more familiar sciences and religions, has ways of opening doors that allow us to "feel the vastness" in new and consequential ways.

In taking up questions of science and religion, knowledge and faith, even truth, beauty, and the good, I stand on the shoulders of giants—including some who have offered Terry Lectures in the past. I think first of Joseph Needham, who spoke at Yale in 1934 as a biochemist, critic of positivism, and almost religious believer in "organicism," at a time prior to his later engagement with the history of Chinese science.[2] I think also of John Dewey (1933–34), pragmatist and educator, whose Terry Lectures—delivered a year before Needham's—form a companion to William James's even earlier lectures in Boston. It is from those latter comments that I draw the quotation above on the charms of philosophy when it is approached as a field of practice.

There are other Terry Lecturers whose talks have drawn my attention.[3] We should recall Henry Sigerist (Terry Lecturer 1939), a historian and physician, who helped to shift medical history from professional biomedical self-congratulation to a globally comparative history of healing (much of it "religious"). There have also been anthropologists like Margaret Mead, Clifford Geertz, and Mary Douglas, each of them bringing a different relativizing approach to the universals sought by previous studies of science and religion. And there have been historical scholars of Asian religions, Donald Lopez (2008) and Wendy Doniger (2014), who have taught anthropologists much about interrogating faiths and reading other worlds. I could also mention Paul Ricoeur (1961–62) and Barbara Herrnstein Smith (2006), who have been influential in anthropology and science studies. Above all, though, the interesting and sustained engagement of this annual lecture series at Yale with concepts of science and religion encouraged me to reengage with American pragmatism. Indeed, Huang Jitang, my principal advisor when I was doing dissertation fieldwork in Guangzhou in the early 1980s, whose curiosity and enthusiasms haunt the discussions of Chinese medicine in this book, considered himself to be an indirect student of John Dewey's, having studied philosophical pragmatism in Hong Kong before 1949.

But rather than further populate this introductory essay with all the giants on whose shoulders I stand, I want to begin by recalling Joseph Needham in particular. His philosophical, philological, and historical approach to the deep history of science in China developed some years after he gave the Terry Lectures in 1934. He died in 1995 after devoting five decades to producing the most influential volumes in the huge and authoritative *Science and Civilisation in China*. His work remains the obligatory starting point for anyone undertaking research that considers culture, technics, and philosophy in the long span of East Asian history.

Joseph Needham was a contentious thinker. Even in his thirties, he was ahead of his time, when as a biochemist he was one of the youngest scholars to deliver the Terry Lectures. His scientific work at the time was especially concerned with the morphogenesis of organisms.[4] And as a historian of science and of China— which is the path he took after the outbreak of the world war in East Asia—he was never more controversial than when he declared Chinese knowledge systems of the past to be *science*. Needham's massive multi-volume *Science and Civilisation in China* project began to see the light of day from Cambridge University Press in the 1950s. He was one among a mid-twentieth-century cohort of path-breaking historians and sociologists of science (one thinks of Robert Merton, George Sarton, John Desmond Bernal, Georges Canguilhem, Ludwik Fleck, Gaston Bachelard, and, later, Thomas Kuhn). The work of these men concatenated to relativize and historicize the truths of science. They made scientific fact social, if no less true. Michel Foucault, further, relying especially on historian of medicine and biology Georges Canguilhem, expanded the field in which truth and knowledge could be not only placed within social practice but profoundly historicized.[5] By showing that rational and objective knowledge is contingent on the human and collective work of producing and configuring facts, these historians showed that European and "Western" science was not just a progressive development from error to truth, from darkness to light, but that science had a history and truth had a social life.[6] In a variety of ways, they showed that the history of truth was not just a triumphal march forward toward ever more perfect representations of a single physical reality. (Working at least a generation later, sociologist John Law has recently started calling this form of science the study of "the one-world world.")[7] In the comparative histories these historians of science undertook, pre-modern physics, chemistry, astronomy, and mathematics in Europe could be shown to be analogous to parallel branches of knowledge and practice in historical East Asia, even though this world region had for so long been thought of as the home not of fact and objectivity but of religion, magic, and mysticism. A comparative or world history of knowledge quickly demonstrated that there had been more than one kind of progress, more than one world to be comprehended.[8] Indeed, in the comparisons Joseph Needham himself undertook, the Chinese sciences sometimes came out looking more "advanced" *as science* than the systems of knowledge contemporary with them in Europe.[9]

I met Joseph Needham and his frequent collaborator Lu Gwei-Djen in the late 1980s, when I enjoyed a brief research stay at the Needham Research Institute in Cambridge. I took the opportunity to ask Professor Lu about the status of their proposed volume 6 on the history of medicine and biology in China.[10] By that time, Lu and Needham had demonstrated great sensitivity to the Chinese sources in a number of fields and time periods, and they had developed not only an encyclopedic grasp of Chinese intellectual history but also a characteristic approach to translation and to the ongoing problem of defining the scientific. They were setting the world standard for scholarship and authoritative critical research in the history of knowledge outside Europe. Their very thorough investigations had identified a number of pre-modern sciences and currents of expertise in East Asia,[11] and their books had begun to revolutionize world opinion about "Chinese civilization." Not entirely immune to Orientalist turns of phrase, the Needham project nevertheless helped the world to appreciate that there had been complex scientific and technological development recorded in the great literature traditions of Asia.

When I met with Professor Lu, very little had appeared in *Science and Civilisation* on the huge topic of medicine and pharmacy, even though I knew this area was near to Lu Gwei-Djen's heart and expertise. She was, after all, the daughter of a Chinese pharmacist (who was, like all herbalists, also a practitioner of Chinese medicine), and her earlier training was in biochemistry. Like Needham, she was likely a committed organicist. Sitting with Dr. Lu in her office, I asked how long we would have to wait for the authoritative English-language history of medicine in China.[12] Dr. Lu shook her head: "Maybe it will never be done," she said. What was the problem? "Chinese medicine," she lamented, "is untranslatable."

I could sympathize, having just written in English my own extended study of the practice of modern Chinese medicine, and having found all translation systems somewhat wanting. But my problems were not quite the same as hers. Dr. Lu and Joseph Needham were suffering from a particular malady brought on by their own historiographical and epistemological convictions. Ultimately, they had faith in the universal truth represented by the modern sciences, and as a result they translated in a way that relied heavily on English-language scientific terms in their translations. This orientation is evident in a "State of the Project" report published about 1980, which predicted that the medicine volume would focus on categories of medical knowledge like diagnosis and prognosis, diseases, immunology, neurology, and otorhinolaryngology. Though these headings for sections appear common sense enough, all could be seen as "bad translations" of historical Chinese medical practices and of comparable terms in Chinese. The report did include a promise that "acupuncture and cautery (moxa)" would receive their own major section; Needham and Lu had already published on this Asia-specific field of therapeutics in 1980.[13] But even the structure of this never-to-be completed volume of *Science and Civilisation* reveals that, in translators' lingo, the source language was pre-modern Chinese "beliefs" and the target language was a refined modern English "science."

I hasten to assure you that Joseph Needham and Lu Gwei-Djen produced some of the most sensitive and respectful readings of pre-modern Chinese thought that we have in the English-language literature. Volume 2, *History of Scientific Thought,* remains a major resource for all of us who try to engage philology, metaphysics, aesthetics, and the unique cultural meanings that inhabit the Chinese language archive. The accounts of Chinese worlds of knowledge and practice to be found in *Science and Civilisation* are nothing if not nuanced, brave, and profoundly honest. But when you examine the very categories in which Needham and his earliest collaborators worked, and the classification schemes that structured their vast assemblage of historical facts, it is clear that their aim as historians of Chinese science was rather determinedly Eurocentric and modernist: if the Chinese classics were to yield a history of *science,* it was ultimately necessary to carve away the superstitious accretions of Chinese religion and cosmology and reveal those kernels of scientific truth—twentieth-century scientific facts—that could be found in the classics, while at the same time rather drastically reorganizing East Asian historical systems—or currents—of thought. This was ultimately a kind of evolutionary history or "progress of knowledge" approach. It has been much discussed as "The Needham Question."[14] And Lu Gwei-Djen was right to think of the difficulty of comprehending Chinese medicine as a *translation* problem, one that especially afflicted medicine. This problem very much troubled her (and probably Joseph Needham too) at the end of their lives.[15]

Translation is a central problem for me as well. Indeed, having spent a fair amount of time reading the critical literature on translation and its general traitorousness, I am inclined to agree with those in the many fields that place translation at the center of their concerns: it is often pointed out that translation is impossible, yet, amazingly, it is happening all the time (see box 1). And at the risk of over-reading Lu Gwei-Djen's lament, I have found in my own work with Chinese medicine that "translation problems" have deep roots in particular philosophical commitments. My differences with the Needham project are philosophical at root and stubborn: I cannot share Needham's deep commitment to the epistemological superiority of modern science and his vision of the evolution of world knowledge toward better and better accounts of only one world.

And this is where we approach the themes of the Terry Lectures, and the real beginning of my own talks on things, thought, and human action. Based on my long engagement as an anthropologist with traditional Chinese medicine, I want to suggest that medicine—all medicine—is a special case of the relations between religion—whatever that is—and science—whatever that is. Many have argued that

Box 1. In Translation: The Needham
Question Expanded

It is common to introduce discussions of the conceptual problems bedeviling all efforts to translate with the Italian adage *traduttore, traditore*: translator, traitor. Certainly, Needham and Lu's modern scientific orientation led to a certain betrayal of the Chinese language of the classical doctors. Terms in Chinese for modern medical things (hormones, sinuses, microbes, spinal column, and so on) had been invented for technical use in modern East Asia by the 1950s, and they could presumably have been projected back into the historical archive to organize the biological insights of "traditional" medicine. Such modern terms could be used to prepare these ideas, as it were, for translation. But the modern terms did not satisfy Dr. Lu's historical style of reading the classic literature. She understood the archive too well on its *own* terms; the referents of biomedical terms were too remote from what Chinese medical experts thought about and acted on over many centuries.

In the *Science and Civilisation* project there was, in addition, a parallel troubled search for anatomical and biodynamic neologisms in Western languages for many terms appearing in pre-modern Chinese that clearly had no English-language equivalents. Understandably, Dr. Lu was reluctant to make Chinese medicine's facts look completely illusory or fantastic through some kind of clunky—or worse, in her eyes, quasi-religious—translation. Perhaps most of all, Needham and Lu reacted against making Chinese knowledge look like magic, religion, or superstition—they were, after all, contributing to the history of *science*.

Dr. Lu didn't discuss this with me at the time we met, but we were all particularly challenged by Chinese medicine's non-anatomical things: not just Qi and its pathways in bodies, but also the life gate

continued

and the triple burner, functional systems that can be spoken of like internal organs but which cannot be found by any dissector or anatomical pathologist. Such entities are easy enough to acknowledge and deploy when one is reading the Chinese sources; they are almost impossible to see as natural objects when we refer to them with English words. And where would science be without object-ivity? It certainly would not be modern![a]

Reflecting on Lu Gwei-Djen's lament, that Chinese medicine is untranslatable, and considering that traditional Chinese medicine (TCM) has now been "translated" around the world, some broad understanding of translation itself would seem to be an essential first step in addressing the relations between science and religion now and in the past. It would be very tempting to analyze Needham and Lu's project in detail as an object lesson in the promises and perils of translating science between worldviews and regimes of practice. This might be a rather discouraging critical project, however. No one wants to be a traitor to a coherent world of truth and healing. Perhaps when Lu Gwei-Djen told me that Chinese medicine is untranslatable, she was expressing her own unwillingness to betray the true meanings of Chinese medical terms, ideas, and practices. The risk was too great that she would be forced to translate perfectly respectable signifiers in Chinese wrongly into the words of a foreign language, killing their life as parts of changing worlds of speech and action.

It is becoming conventional, however, at least in my field, to point out that translation is not simply a matter of converting "languages" into each other, tidying away words and meanings, dealing only with concepts as we go. The mentalist biases of a model of language that presumes an exchange between conceiving minds (while leaving bodies and worlds in brackets) have come in for considerable critique and recasting in anthropology.[b] In the place of communication we tend to speak of circulations, traffic, transfer, transduction. And in all these mobilities we try to take note of concomitant transformations, which is to say, transmutations not just of words on pages but of forms of life, alterations in the very nature of things. Everything changes as it goes: information is translated and "transcribed" between proteins in molecular biology. Evidence is translated between laboratory benches and bedsides in community hospitals. Institutional forms from American government agencies are taken up and recast to fit new circumstances in so-called developing countries. Things or entities once seen as quite fixed become novel "matters of concern" in always historically specific situations. And the translations attempted in ethnography are intrinsically political. Post-colonial studies have insisted on recognizing the stubborn asymmetries of power and value attaching to languages as they play out and inter-transform in real worlds.[c]

Once translation has become a matter of the transfer and transformation of entities, forces, and agents (and concepts too) between partly commensurable or not entirely inconceivable worlds, we can see more easily that nothing goes untranslated: translation is always already going on, even deep within language worlds identified as the same. We can hardly help trying to translate, if we want to connect and communicate beyond some solipsistic half-existence riddled with doubt. Any ethnographer with experience working in a second language—like me—has ruefully noticed the ongoing problem of what I, doing field research in rural southern China, came to call "infra-translation": struggling as a foreigner to understand what's being said, one notices similar struggles among "the natives." "What? Say that again? Who did you say you saw? Sorry, I forgot." How often do we hear such utterances over our own dinner tables, in elevators, over the phone?

Translating, we continually face failure: too often, the "right translation," sought by, among others, Arthur Waley, is simply not to be

continued

had.[d] Perhaps it is as we engage the highly various practices of translation that we see the pragmatic imperative most clearly: for the critical humanities, disciplining our words and concepts is not enough, and full communication is an ever-receding goal.

And yet, we keep struggling toward the right phrasing, the telling image, the formation that truly captures and clarifies and conveys something other and different. We are thrilled when we find that unfamiliar thing that travels well. One such traveling reality might be that classic field of shared significance, "the body." The body as anatomically structured container of an abstract individual is not the universal foundation of human existence it is often thought to be. But lived bodies—like the form of embodiment brought forth and made salient in a medical practice—are full of surprises. When we embark on the translation of Chinese medical things, thought, and action into the experience of sufferers, new and marvelous worlds emerge.[e] This book aims to read some of those unexpected worlds through language.

a. Daston and Galison, *Objectivity*.

b. See Sapir, "Unconscious Patterning of Behavior." Somewhat more indirect materialist approaches to language, also relatively early, include Bakhtin, "Discourse in the Novel," and Foucault, *Order of Things*.

c. Latour, *Inquiry into Modes of Existence*. For post-colonial translation, see Asad, "Concept of Cultural Translation," and Niranjana, *Siting Translation*. Niranjana emphasizes the disruptive potential of translation, an orientation close to the aims of this book. See also Liu, *Translingual Practice*. I am indebted for some of my phrasing here to Professor Susan Gal, who has inspired much thinking about translation at the University of Chicago.

d. On Arthur Waley, see Morris, ed., *Madly Singing in the Mountains*.

e. Acupuncturist Cinzia Scorzon has recently been asking her patients in follow-up interviews to articulate in words their sensations and responses during treatment. The experiences reported by this diverse group are full of surprises for anyone (like most of us) who tends to take for granted a commonsense modernist body. See Zhan, *Other-Worldly*, for a parallel use of "worlding" as a verb relevant to Chinese medicine.

clinical medicine, because it is so practical and full of nasty surprises, or uncontrolled variables, should not be thought of as a science in itself. The laboratory is relatively remote from the clinic. This we increasingly know, as whole groups of clinicians and hospital administrators wrangle the complexities of transporting knowledge "from bench to bedside" in the new biomedical specialty of "translational medicine." Every clinician also knows that effective healing requires more than the mechanical application of scientific knowledge to never-uniform human bodies. Moreover, though "faith in the healer" has often been invoked to explain some of the little miracles that take place in any medical setting, most modern scholars reject the idea that faith alone can heal the real illnesses recognized in any therapeutic system. So medicine is not only not a science, it is not a religion either.[16]

Nathan Sivin—one of my inspiring teachers—has been known to say that medicine is everywhere more an art or craft than a science, more a cultural formation than a natural science.[17] This can be said of all kinds of medicine, including folk medicines from all over the world, the kinds of cultural forms that interested Henry Sigerist in his 1939 Terry Lectures. When I have tried this idea out on well-educated, scientifically inclined users of Western biomedicine in China, they have embraced the idea, no doubt thinking of the many uncertainties in play (e.g., about causes, see appendix 1) in even the most advanced clinical settings, and hoping that their doctors are not only aware of the latest science and using the best technology but also, and especially, that they are perceptive, imaginative, artful, and attentive to the particular situation at hand. This notion that medicine is at heart an art, albeit one that draws on both science and faith, invites us to understand world medicine with methods drawn from aesthetics or poetics. But I worry that such subtle approaches might trivialize or marginalize a seldom beautiful but nevertheless deeply serious collective undertaking: every style of medicine that addresses human suffering with the best tools at hand.

But let me return to the challenge offered by the Terry Lectures on the relations between science and religion, and insist now that medicine is the field of human endeavor that most challenges the idea that religion and science are different things. As I was preparing these lectures in August 2018, I opened the morning paper to find an advertisement for a "One Day University" event in which a biologist from Brown University, Kenneth Miller, was scheduled to deliver a lecture titled "Religion vs. Science: Forever in Conflict?" This confirmed me in my determination to demonstrate that science and religion are not so different. It is not Professor Miller's science, or his religion, that I might like to challenge—though of course I didn't know what he planned to say—but rather that little "versus" that is conventionally put between them.[18] I hope to show you in a variety of ways that anthropological observation and our disciplinary orientation to practice suggest that *pragmatically* there is no essential difference between science and religion, any more than a radical empiricism à la William James can find a defining difference between thing and thought.[19] After the historians and sociologists of science, after Joseph Needham and other comparativists, we are no longer presented with two looming terms between which a relationship must be forged. Many of us have a downright religious commitment to the idea that biomedicine as it is practiced in our academic medical centers is scientific, and a parallel conviction that every other healing modality is somehow religious. In our core curricula, as in our public culture, the scientific essence of biomedicine and the superstitious heart of "culture" are both taken on faith. Structurally, moreover, we sort things apart: we are content to have most sorts of confessed faith managed in the hospital chaplain's office and the divinity school, or perhaps referred to the psychiatry ward. Meanwhile, clinicians are encouraged to lean on a statistical "evidence base" in the expectation that quantitative science will reduce the uncertainty of their actions. This, despite the fact that evidence, these days, is most often expressed as probabilities, not causal certainties. In these institutionalized commitments to the difference and distance between religion and science, we are the heirs of that long twentieth-century philosophical project of secularizing truth, the great work of positivist epistemology that drew a boundary between scientific objectivity and the religious domain of metaphysics, cultural beliefs, ultimate meanings, and spiritual life. But we do not need to capitulate to the compartmentalization of kinds of truth that positivism reinforced, nor do we have to wring our hands over that little "versus" that is so often inserted between religion and science.

When it is looked at from the point of view of any non-Euro-American form of systematic knowledge, when it is studied comparatively as historians and sociologists began to do long ago, science in practice—especially in clinics, but also in laboratories—reveals its "superstitious" and "magical" character. The unproven metaphysical assumptions that underlie any physics, the philosophical rationalist's insistence on the universality of certain fundamental categories like space, time, matter, and spirit (so wonderfully critiqued by William James and other radical empiricists): these are not necessary conditions of all human thought and knowledge. Rather they are specific cultural-religious commitments that, as Emile Durkheim demonstrated in *The Elementary Forms of the Religious Life* over one hundred years ago, are socially constructed. Because social formations have varied so much, and because both knowledge and belief, science and religion, are constituted in highly diverse social practices, we have inherited a plural universe that invites us to learn from differences, in depth, as philosophers.

My use of that pesky pronoun "we" in these pages deserves some comment at the outset. Who is it to whom I address lectures like these? Who is that reader who might be confronted with deeply unfamiliar things, thoughts, and actions in a book about Chinese medicine? How does "difference" appear as different from what we—this group includes me as author—always thought was common sense? The answer to these questions has to do with my commitment to translation (see box 1). Translators of technical knowledge systems know this well: even with the massive mixtures and hybrids, technology transfers and modernizations that have resulted from several hundred years of cultural and linguistic globalization, there are a great many stubbornly local things to which "foreign" words refer. Rather than betray the local uniqueness of these referents, these "things," it sometimes feels right in a translation process to embrace their strangeness. That anglophone world that reads the Terry Lectures may balk at some of the un-smooth, nonidiomatic ideas and images that appear in Chinese medical writing. Appendix 2 of this volume contains some lovely examples of entities and processes that do not work in the "one-world world" critiqued by John Law. I know from confusing experience that "we," that loose collectivity for whom the English language naturally refers to a commonsense world, have much to learn.

We learn from differences as philosophers, certainly, but we also learn as vulnerable bodies and conscientious actors. Today's shrinking world offers more and more opportunities to feel the problematic thrill of thinking otherwise. With these Terry Lectures I seek to recruit you to a reading of the writings and practices of traditional Chinese medicine for yourselves, to invite you to make a place in your mind for the things, thought, and action of a non-Western medicine and style of thought. In what follows, I devote chapter 2 to defining and describing some of the *things* with which Chinese doctors work in the clinics where they see and effectively treat a great many patients. These things—qi, circulation tracks, powerful flavors, functional organs like the triple burner or the life gate—have been controversial in global health discourses, but I will argue that they are just as real, or unreal, as a thyroid gland, immunity, metabolism, or pathogenic stress.[20] It is precisely in the domain of things, the beings that are specific to a Chinese medical world, that a certain battle for the truth is being fought. This is especially true in the United States, where I am constantly being told that the entities addressed by Chinese medical experts are ridiculous or fantastic, not scientifically valid. Chapter 2, on things, suggests that it is not a greater acceptance of fantasy that is required, but rather an expanded materialism, a fuller appreciation of concrete practice, which can make sense of qi transformation and the circulatory body.

Chapter 3 develops examples of the modes of reasoning that could be called the thought style of modern traditional Chinese medicine, or TCM. Revisiting some of my own earlier treatments of the "knowing practice" of modern Chinese medicine,[21] I reintroduce the logic of TCM's clinical encounter, dwelling on modes of perception, discernment of patterns, and the quest for insight into the sources of manifest symptoms. Chapter 3 also explores "correlative thought," which though far from unknown in the Euro-American traditional sciences, has in China been developed as a form of medical reasoning founded on an ancient yet still useful understanding of ontogenesis. That is to say, the scientific puzzle of morphogenesis—how living entities reliably emerge as particular forms—has a Chinese solution (albeit one that can never answer all the interesting questions, just as molecular genetics cannot). This discussion draws on the work of contemporary doctors of Chinese medicine to insist that their way of thinking about the roots and sources of the living forms that are manifest all round us is *useful.* Doctors using Chinese medical means to treat disease often remind themselves that they should trace a very particular root. How they do this is a fascinating technical matter, taken up in part in chapter 4.

Chapter 4 considers the practical consequences and ethical commitments of the work that must be done in a world populated by suffering bodies, disputed things, powerful medicines, and unreliable stabs at rational explanation. Medical practitioners of all kinds are valued because they have an unusual expertise: they can see in a way that allows them to infer the invisible,[22] their experience helps them to think their way toward wise prognosis, and their tool kit includes relatively harmless ways to alter the sufferings of those who seek their help. Medicine is an ethical undertaking in several senses of the word. One irreducible part of this medical ethics is the effort made by any practitioner to grasp the experience of another person in order to nudge his or her organic process in more wholesome directions. How do healers sort through the ethical and technical imperatives that guide their lives of service? How should we, for that matter?

Chinese medicine can show us a world known and treated by a healing art both ancient and modern, both mundane and philosophical. By the end of this book, I aim to clarify a Chinese medical approach to action in general, not solely the action of healing. Rather, we can reflect on action in a world of not entirely visible things and processes that are not easy to understand, requiring clarity of mind and acceptance of the reality of some invisible but powerful things. I urge attention to Chinese medicine not because it will directly or immediately improve health and relieve suffering—though it does do these things around the world—but because this ever-changing body of knowledge can give us the problematic thrill of thinking deep things in translation. It can help us to feel the presence of the vastness. William James believed that that opening is valuable in itself; so do I.

2

Things: Myriad and Gathering

The great vacuity cannot be without qi.
Qi cannot but gather, thus to become the myriad things.
The myriad things cannot but scatter,
thus to become the great vacuity.

Zhang Zai, eleventh century, *Correcting Ignorance*[1]

Let's begin with *things*. "The Thing" is a stubbornly massy problem of both epistemology and ontology. It keeps renewing itself as a
question in modern philosophy, comparative anthropology, and cultural history. Heidegger, in his fascinating essay "The Thing," uses
a humble water jug as an example of a thing that is gathered into
salient ("present at hand") existence for the philosopher on whose
desk it sits.[2] He challenges us to place this most solid, concrete, and
ordinary object, this usually ignored thing, into its specific history
of making, serving, and being used (sometimes even as an example
of thing-hood). Other materialist philosophers have made the classic
schoolroom gesture toward chairs and tables,[3] asking pupils to re-
experience them as problematic and imagine a world that is perhaps
not so solidly given as they commonsensibly think. The Chinese
metaphysical tradition has used the term "the myriad (or 10,000)
things" (*wanwu* 万物) as a term for phenomenal reality itself, and

many philosophical discussions have relied on this phrase to remind anglophone readers of classic texts in translation that the material world (*wu*, concrete things) is vast, plural, and hard to pin down (*wan*, or myriad, teeming).[4] Bruno Latour and Peter Weibel remind us that the very word "thing" derives from a history of political assembly in Europe, *das Ding*, a gathering.[5] Their observation reminds us that even the most self-evident objects have a history of "social construction."

Objects and things have lately been star performers in our more philosophically inclined classrooms, as a fresh turn toward metaphysics and "object oriented ontology" inspires renewed speculation on the nature of materiality.[6] But medicine offers us even more interesting entities than these classroom examples, things that we can both appreciate in their stubborn materiality and test in our own experience. Medical things, as I will show throughout this essay, are real in their consequences.[7] And where illness and healing are concerned, consequences are both hard to foresee and very substantial.

Qi, Substance, Activity

The thing belonging to Chinese medicine that most often stops a translator cold is *qi* 气／氣. It has been rendered in English as configurative energy (Porkert), pneuma (Lu and Needham), or vital energy (cf. Kaptchuk), but most recent translators have preferred to leave the word untranslated. We struggle to come up with metaphors and descriptions that can explain the complexity of this thing—if qi is a thing—to our students and English-speaking friends.[8] Everyone hesitates before the impossibility of defining this most basic actor in the Chinese medical cosmos. Those of us who write about traditional Chinese medicine (TCM) in translation have mostly found that we have no choice but to accept the existence of qi, in all its reality and power, in its irreducible plurality *and* its utter simplicity.[9]

The "meaning" of "qi" has not just been a problem for those of us who traffic in words and things as we translate between language worlds. Though most of the history of Chinese philosophy has seen the word used as a commonsense noun, no more in need of definition than air or water, time, space, or substance, there have been moments in the history of Chinese thought when "qi" has been problematized.[10] Zhang Zai, for example, quoted in this chapter's epigraph, undertook considerable reflection on the nature and propensities of qi in his metaphysical writings. In doing so, he was reviving a broadly metaphysical moment in East Asian thought and politics, about one thousand years after the classical age, and like his philosophical ancestors he was reconsidering fundamental categories at a time of rapid social change.[11]

Jumping forward another one thousand years, we can see that the modern scholar-doctors who were tasked with sorting and systematizing TCM for a swiftly expanding institutional life, in the renaissance moment of China's 1980s, also had to concern themselves with the proper definitions of elusive entities going by ancient names, such as qi.[12] Some of this work on the meanings of words was required as glosses of key terms in reference works like dictionaries, clinical handbooks, and introductory textbooks. Ideally, for these modern systematizers, all of the famous ambiguity of classical Chinese words would be channeled into tidily structured concepts, and words like "qi" would refer to straightforwardly empirical things.[13] Given the size and contentiousness of the philosophical archive, this was not a job for the faint of heart! "Qi" is, after all, a very ancient term and—for anyone with an education—its meanings draw on the far from identical visions of many philosophies. Moreover, among experts, much of the enjoyment of working with things like qi arises from the very productive indeterminacy of such notions, as they have appeared in so many different literatures over so many hundreds of years.[14]

A textbook edited by Deng Tietao in the early 1980s preserves a sense of the difficulty. Here is his paragraph opening the chapter on "Qi, Blood, Fluids":

> *Qi* is the basic material making up the human body, and it is one of the material bases of the life activity of the human body. At the same time, the ancients also called all the manifest forms of the various life activities of the human body qi. Founded on this recognition, the qi spoken of in TCM is conceptualized as two senses of the word: One is the essential subtle matter that composes and sustains the life activity of the human body. It is an ever active (*yundongzhede* 运动着的) infinitesimal and imperceptible mobile nutritive substance, e.g., the qi of food and water, or the qi that is breathed. The second sense of the word indicates the functional physiology of the visceral structures, e.g., the qi of the five yin visceral systems, the qi of the six yang visceral systems, the qi that flows in the circulation tracks, etc. But these two meanings are interconnected, the former qi is the material basis of the latter qi, and the latter is the functional expression of the former.[15]

This way of setting up qi for students and future clinicians admits that the modern dual characterization of this ancient thing (echoed in many sources since the definitional moment of the late 1970s and early 1980s) is a limitation imposed on a richly ambiguous ancient term: qi is *now conceptualized* as substance and action at once. This is a terminological discussion, and "qi" might as well appear between quotation marks (as it was appearing in a great deal of philosophical and medical literature at the time, in fact). But its reality is unquestioned. Here, qi is matter and action, and these two are inseparable in a qi-composed universe: matter enables configured activity, activity expresses configurations of matter. Already an ontological hybrid, at least in "Western" terms, the meaning of qi is not much narrowed by Deng Tietao's technical definition. A dictionary definition, also from 1982, demonstrates the breadth of the thing even more clearly: "Qi: The most basic material entity forming the myriad things of the universe. . . . Qi is divided as yin and yang, suggesting the unification of substance and function, as well as reminding us of principles by which the myriad things are transformed from qi."[16] Both definitions are tautologies: the material activity called qi, we are reassured, precisely is nothing other than material and active. This is not a failure of thinking, it is an entry into the ontological. The thing itself evades definition.

But qi can be known in experience, beyond all bookish fine points. Acupuncturists and their patients "get qi" (*de qi* 得气) routinely in therapeutic practice. Cinzia Scorzon, a practitioner who teaches acupuncture at Westminster University (London), in a recent essay describes the event of getting qi as follows: "*De qi* is a sensation experienced by patients and acupuncturists after needle insertion, a sensible response that connects the needle and the pathways of the body."[17] In her expert description of a routine clinical reality, Scorzon insists on both the materiality of qi (it is "sensible") and its character as a form of activity (it is a "response that connects").[18] She is aware, of course, that some readers of her study will be skeptical of this unscientific "thing," qi. She goes on to reassure us:

How do I know that qi has arrived? I perceive that something has grasped the sharp end of the needle below the surface, at times I feel a mild electrical current coming from below to my fingers. The patient's breathing changes and becomes deeper, and peristaltic noises might occur.[19]

In Scorzon's account, qi is something that happens to the practitioner, the patient, and the needles that link them as bodies.

In her research with patients, Scorzon collected a number of fascinating articulations of experience while being needled. None of her interviewees had read the "theory" of qi circulation or knew about Chinese medical pathways of the body. Yet they reported concrete events that accorded exactly with a technical TCM understanding of the flow of qi. For Scorzon and others, this is *tong* 通, through-passage.[20] "Most interviewees," she says, "experienced something tangible going through and connecting various parts of their body: they experienced *tong*." In their words, qi was "something like a current," "a fuzzy bubbling sensation," "a surge of energy coming up my body."[21] The way in which qi's forcefulness and mobility work throughout the body was noted by some patients: "I became aware of different parts of my body I was not aware of before"; "I feel very aware of every part of the body, including the ears and toes."[22] And, as Scorzon notes, some patients waxed poetic or conceptual: acupuncture produces "a feeling of warmth spreading in my body, with a feeling of returning; something I missed has come back." Or, "the treatment reassembles me, everything seems to go back to where it is supposed to be, the right place."[23]

Experienced in these ways, qi does not lend itself to being acknowledged as a mere thing, especially if we use the English word "thing" in its usual clunky sense. Rather, as Zhang Zai points out (see this chapter's epigraph), "qi cannot but gather . . . to become the myriad things." Gathering is a process, not an object; but this process is no less real than the objects it throws up or allows us to "get."

Ontological Disease

Here's another problematic and important example of thing-hood, this time from the history of biomedicine: "ontological disease." The identification, classification, and eradication of diseases as such, especially acute infectious diseases, in individual "cases" or in populations, are hallmark tasks of modern biomedicine. In the nineteenth and twentieth centuries, disease became a kind of *thing*. It emerged with the rise of pathological anatomy, and later bacteriology, as a privileged entity demanding to be perceived and understood by physicians. Yet as Ludwik Fleck pointed out quite brilliantly in 1935, even a fairly well-understood disease like syphilis had to be painstakingly assembled by rather contentious thought collectives: syphilis was gathered together in recognizable, diagnosable form as a convergence of symptoms, laboratory test results, drug responsiveness, and clinician-researchers who were trained and who related to each other in historically specific ways.[24] Even today, this disease is not definable through reduction to presence or absence of a single bacterium, since many who are exposed to *Treponema pallidum pallidum* actually do not develop a "case" of the disease.

Yet no one (least of all Fleck) challenges the reality of syphilis — if we put the problem of its thing-hood in pragmatist terms, the entity syphilis is a very convenient, indeed supremely serviceable, *thing*. Diagnosed, it can be distinguished from (or carved away from, known apart from — this is what diagnosis means) the confusing, excessive, and rather particular discomforts of its human host. *It* can be *treated*, using an antibiotic like penicillin that seeks out and disrupts the most vulnerable element in the assemblage that is syphilis, that point of interruption being the bacterium. And, like the qi that flows through and unites the bodies of Cinzia Scorzon's acupuncture patients, this antibiotic is no respecter of persons: it works whether or not the sufferer has faith in it or even knows what sort of a thing it is. Syphilis is not just a figment of someone's imagination (nor is qi);[25] rather it is an insistent interlocutor of human experts and refined pharmaceuticals in clinical settings.

But the very actuality of ontological disease in biomedicine has been a problem for a modernizing and globalizing Chinese medicine. This "traditional Chinese medicine" is a field that analyzes physical disorders mostly without relying on those biomedical technologies that can visualize lesions or quantify microbial invaders hidden inside bodies. Chinese medicine acts on disease without collecting the kinds of "objective" information that is invisible to the naked eye but obtainable through sample extraction and microscopy, like white cell counts or PSI levels, for example. Of course, these apparent gaps are troublesome: caught up in an obsessive modernist orientalism that insists on comparing China to the West, medical system to medical system, TCM can only appear as backward and lacking. But practitioners of Chinese medicine are conversant with a vast literature recording and critically evaluating hundreds of years of notably effective healing experience, and most of them are not willing to see their knowledge as falling short or being fundamentally in error. Yet they must practice in a world where syphilis, for example, is an uncontestable *thing* even though they have no history of diagnosing and treating it as a discrete ontological disease.

Let's step back a bit and reflect on how the challenge of a biomedical ontology has been received in modern China. From at least the 1920s forward, there have been challenges by modernizers to (what came to be thought of as) the "theory" of Chinese medicine.[26] Many argued that the only part of the field that should be retained in a modern health services system was the effective materia medica, which could be used together with science and technology taken from "the West." Materia medica, note, could be imagined as a comfortably commonsense collection of objects—plants, animal parts, some minerals—each with certain "active properties," many of which would be good candidates for relatively simple addition into the pharmacopeia of biomedicine. Meanwhile, the "theory," all the putatively superstitious lore premised on Chinese medicine's living body of flow and transformations,[27] could safely be scuttled in the interest of building a truly modern and scientific China. The efforts of these scientifically educated citizens of China to adopt the same ontological character—and the same collection of commonsense objects—as the rest of the scientific one-world world were part of a thoroughly political project: modernization and development under the guidance of the emergent and embattled nation-state.

Fortunately for the growth of Chinese medicine in China, the abolitionist position never fully succeeded, and as we know, in the 1950s the People's Republic of China established the first officially pluralist national health and medicine system in the world.[28] In 1956, Mao Zedong declared traditional medicine in China to be a "great treasure-house" and started to delineate a policy of expansion, modernization, and regulation of the field. The rapid growth of traditional medicine institutions in the 1950s and '60s, and then again in the 1980s after the end of the cultural revolution decade, returned a number of "traditional" practitioners to local and national prominence. These leaders formed curriculum committees, wrote textbooks and reference works, collected herbal prescriptions and case histories (in the millions), and taught vast numbers of medical students how to think and heal with a newly systematized TCM.[29] These were the experienced experts who needed to come to terms with, and sometimes resist, the ontological diseases known to "Western" biomedicine.

Pattern of Disorder

In the context of this medical revolution, what did TCM propose in place of biomedical things like syphilis? In other words, lacking technologies of diagnosis that could strip illness to its essentials for instant intervention (in the way that penicillin can eradicate *Treponema pallidum pallidum* without worrying about all the other causal factors and conditions determining presence or absence of "syphilis"), how does TCM "know apart," or diagnose? Is there a TCM nosology, or list of officially recognized diseases? How does the Chinese doctor give a name—an actionable name, linkable to therapeutic procedures—to what is happening in the suffering body?

These two "Western medical," or biomedical, hallmarks, the disease and the diagnosis, were under intensive discussion when I began my field research in a college of traditional Chinese medicine in southern China in the early 1980s. I have written elsewhere about this renaissance moment for the field, so I will not belabor the debates here.[30] Instead we can examine the terms that came to stand in for disease and diagnosis, as Chinese medicine developed in a tense relationship of contrast and resistance alongside the growth of modern biomedical knowledge and service delivery in China.

"Diagnosis," for example, is nicely translated in Chinese as *zhenduanxue* (诊断学), a compound of "examination" and "a cut" or "differentiation"—so, a good rendering of diagnosis as "knowing apart."[31] But mid-century Chinese medical thinkers could not be satisfied with that term, given all its associations with taxonomies and nosologies of "Western" ontological diseases. It did not seem to describe their own most crucial clinical practice of understanding and naming pathological disorder. Instead, over a period of a few years of committee work among a fairly diverse collection of experts, they developed a methodological commitment to *bianzheng lunzhi* (辨证论治), or pattern discernment and therapy determination. This is the logical and practical formation that I analyzed at length in my first book, *Knowing Practice.* Figure 1 is a simplified version of that lengthy representation of the TCM clinical encounter. It diagrams the sequence of logical and co-constructive steps that are supposed to be taken in a standard modern clinical encounter. Reading up and down the sequence, from lower left to lower right, one can

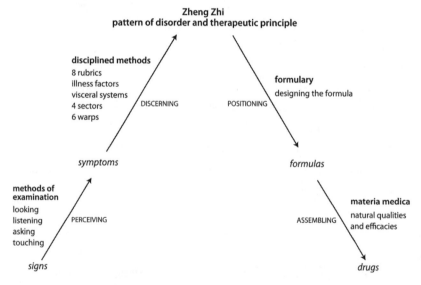

Figure 1. The pattern-discerning and therapy-determining process

see how a pattern of disorder and a drug treatment emerge in medical work.

Working with the "signs" presented by the patient, a doctor uses skilled examination techniques (pulse touching, tongue inspection, history-taking, for example) to generate a list of somewhat medicalized "symptoms" (insomnia, floating pulse, dry mouth, etc.). Symptoms can be understood through a variety of correlational analytic methods (the eight rubrics and the yin and yang visceral systems are examples), and, with the help of these analytic correlations, a pattern of disorder can be perceived and named. The pattern leads to a "therapeutic principle"—an allopathic one, usually, in the sense that an opposing influence is ranged against the tendency of the symptoms (heat against cold, yang against yin), and that therapeutic idea is supposed to guide the careful design, or positioning (*chufang* 处方), of a drug formula. The clinical encounter—in herbal medicine, anyway—culminates in a structured collection of natural medicines ready to boil and swallow as a "soup" (*tang* 汤) or decoction. The materia medica, or collection of things, positioned together in a prescription and gathered in a paper parcel by the pharmacy, once boiled and swallowed, release their healing powers. And they do so in interaction with the pathological process that has been assembled, discerned, and named as a pattern.

Many of my teachers in China felt that *bianzheng lunzhi,* as a practice of knowing illness, grasping the trajectory of symptoms, and intervening in pathological process, amounted to the essential or core technical virtue of their field.[32] As a "style of thought" (*siwei fangshi* 思维方式), this formation summarized their valued expertise and organized their attentiveness in the clinic. *Bianzheng lunzhi* was also a teachable technique: it has structured medical school curricula for TCM with, for example, its distinction between the fields of formulary and pharmaceutics, which came to be taught separately. This disciplined approach to recognizing a pattern—which occupies the top of this diagram and functions as the pivot of the representing and intervening process of the clinical encounter—was felt to encapsulate the virtuoso skill of the experienced doctor.[33]

Why was the "disease" that is "known apart" as a thing by biomedicine replaced in this modern TCM formation with "pattern"? What kind of an entity is a collectively recognized and practically discerned pattern? The Chinese word in use in the 1980s was *zheng* 证 or *zhenghou* 证候. A 1988 dictionary defines *zhenghou* as follows: "What is composed from a set of interconnected symptoms and bodily signs (including tongue image, pulse image, etc.), and reflects certain regularities of illness change."[34] Theorists, including some of those who compiled this dictionary, worked hard to regularize the relationship, both contrasting and overlapping, between disease and pattern. Eventually, during this period of rapid change in knowledge and institutional policies, the two terms, disease (*jibing* 疾病) and pattern (*zhenghou* 证候) were disciplined into a cooperative existence. Every case record was required to have a "Western medicine" disease diagnosis, and in clinics of "Chinese medicine" doctors concentrated on supplementing this diagnosis with a carefully discerned TCM pattern. The result was that in TCM clinics, therapy could proceed on the basis of the pattern, not the diagnosis.[35] At the same time, the "Western medicine" diagnosis allowed relatively easy movement, for the patient at least, between modes of treatment. Mobility of this kind, between clinics and practitioners, is highly valued in China's pluralistic medical system.

But let's look more closely at what a "pattern" is, by way of the dictionary definition quoted above: "What is composed from a set of interconnected symptoms and bodily signs (including tongue image, pulse image, etc.), and reflects certain patterns of illness change." First of all, it is *composed*—though the definition does not say by whom. But the ingredients of which it is composed suggest a particular agency, that of the observant doctor: these interconnected symptoms and bodily signs are *images* legible to the physician, with his trained perception. "Tongue image, pulse image, etc." are *signs* that are read from the surface of the body; and it is an essential part of this reading process (which relies on the doctor's own senses of vision, touch, hearing, etc.) to discover that these images form "an interconnected set." But the set is not out there in wild nature, as an ontological disease, somehow (implausibly) freestanding and unchanging. Patterns come to the clinic one by one, expressed in the individual and idiosyncratic bodies and histories of patients. Following the ontology of Zhang Zai (recalling again this chapter's epigraph) both doctor and patient probably see the *zheng* pattern as already being gathered into a sort of thing-hood that predates its presentation in the clinic. But medicine takes over the composing process, finding a way to express the materiality of the disorder as a pattern that can be treated. This approach to the TCM pattern amounts to pattern recognition, seeing the thing in its integrity but inseparably from its natural habitat, which is to say, the particular human being.

But the key thing that differentiates the expertly composed, or gathered, Chinese medical pattern from ontological disease is that it is not other than its inferred "interconnected set" of concrete *relations*. That is to say, unlike syphilis or cholera, it is not abstracted from the specific clinical situation, it is not thought to exist as a thing in the world, discrete and with fixed attributes, awaiting discovery in diagnosis. Rather like a constellation in which (William James says somewhere) the several stars might be rather surprised, if they were told about it, to find themselves a representation of a human myth,[36] the illness pattern's integrity as a medical thing derives entirely from what can be perceived from a human point of view. It is composed—again and again, in varying ways—in the clinical encounter. It is no wonder that the "great treasure house" of Chinese medicine records thousands of names for *zhenghou*—the pattern is a description of a contingent configuration, even a constellation, not a single official term for a stable, discrete, or autonomous thing.

A pattern is not for all that merely imaginary. It is still a very real and materially manifested thing, as Chinese theorists have argued and daily proved in their clinics. One of my occasional teachers in Guangzhou, for example, Deng Tietao (his definition of qi is cited above), worried that the biomedical entity of disease, in contemporary practice, was overshadowing the Chinese medical notion of pattern. Though Deng wrote an extremely useful handbook called *Practical TCM Diagnosis*, displaying his practical commitment to a biomedical notion of "knowing apart," he was also known as a leading theorist of pattern discernment and therapy determination, that is, of *bianzheng lunzhi*.[37] He did not succumb willingly to the hegemony of a Western medicine object world. Indeed, not long after I first visited his clinic in the 1980s he turned to doing research on the history of Chinese medicine. He seems to have decided that responsible clinical work could not proceed without careful attention to a classical past, and it needed to include respectful recording of a history that revealed plural—if partly lost—worlds.

Another great thinker, Lu Guangxin, whose best philosophy was written during the renaissance of the 1980s, insisted on speaking of the *zhenghou* pattern as a thing. At the same time, he placed "pattern" in strong contrast to the biomedical "disease" that already dominated clinical case records in the 1980s. Explicitly affiliating himself with Maoist materialism and practice epistemology, Lu was far from being a vulgar ontologist of "the thing itself."[38] The word he used for "thing," for example, was thoroughly relational and emergent. His "thing" was a *duixiang* (对象). Translated literally this means "the image we face." (It also means counterpart, target, even romantic partner or fiancé.)[39] Lu Guangxin has no trouble with the idea that an illness pattern, a pattern of disorder, can be treated as an object that is contemplated by an expert knower. He has no problem, either, with the accepted idea that this thing is composed in practice by those who are able to recognize it as a pattern. In fact, he argues that the skilled healer must make certain limiting choices about what to see, what to read, what to note down, what to gather together. To see his point, look again at figure 1: the methods of examination generate medicine-specific "symptoms," which is a smaller set, very often, than the full array of complaints, or the signs brought to the doctor's attention by the patient. "Insomnia" and "many dreams" might be noted as symptoms but not the fact that my dead mother visited me in one of those dreams. The discerner of significant patterns must set priorities—it would be folly to see every manifestation of bodily life as symptomatic, much less as part of an interrelated system. So, difficult decisions must be made, things must be sorted. Some of the myriad things are not salient to modern medicine. (This stance will be discussed at greater length in chapter 4.)

Lu Guangxin writes about things in a Maoist sloganeering idiom that has a chip on its shoulder. His style is highly entertaining, though it was not appreciated by all his colleagues at the University of Traditional Chinese Medicine in Beijing. But Lu is deeply serious in proposing a radically different idea of a thing than a biomedical diagnostician of ontological diseases would be dealing with.[40] Lu writes as if the *duixiang* might be a bit of a scandal, an unacceptable concept to modern bioscience and even to China's national health policy. We should bear in mind that Lu was writing in a climate of relentless comparison between "China" and "the West," especially as post-Mao China was embracing the "four modernizations" and seeking to "get on track with the world." He was part of a group of Chinese medical thinkers who were still trying to preserve the specificity of their field against the generalizing universals propagated in modern biology. The *duixiang*-thing was, I feel, a major contribution.

There was a joking comment current among intellectual and clinical leaders of TCM at the time Dr. Lu was writing about TCM things: "Western medicine knows all about dead bodies, but Chinese medicine understands the *life* of bodies." It is as if they had been reading Foucault! And perhaps, indirectly, they had. Note that the word for anatomy in Chinese, *jiepouxue* (解剖学), translates literally as "dissection study," or the science based on opening up and separating. The concept is very closely related to the "knowing apart" of "diagnosis." Older Chinese doctors, on the other hand, as discerners of processual patterns, readers of the unstable signs that faced them in clinics, saw little use for "Western medical" knowledge about bones, organs, and tissues, which modern biomedicine had developed in the course of its history of dissection and pathological anatomy. A heart or liver that can be cut from its embedding structures in the body, and known as such, as a discrete and static object, is not a human or medical thing for the leaders of modern TCM.

Recall the pragmatic understanding of pattern defined above: a *zhenghou* is "what is composed from a set of interconnected symptoms and bodily signs (including tongue image, pulse image, etc.), and reflects certain patterns of illness change." Patterns are actively *composed* from the signs of life, the symptoms of disorder; they make sense as moments in a process of living change. Theorists like Lu

Guangxin, along with the authors of "Basic Theory of TCM" text-books in the 1980s, as they contrasted the *zheng* pattern with the on-tological disease, were mounting a principled resistance to a scientific assault on their very bodies. They were skilled knowing subjects who had learned, through much hardship and drawing on the effective experience of their forebears and teachers, to discern the patterns of pathology presented by actual living patients under very real material conditions. They could learn anatomy (and younger doctors do), but they couldn't see much use for it.[41]

Organs and Visceral Systems

What is an organ, then? Consider the dis-embedded anatomical organ, cut free and held in the hands of the dissecting pathologist or transplant surgeon. This heart or kidney is certainly an objec-tive thing, it has borders, attributes, a structure. It takes up a certain amount of space. As object, it preexisted its surgical removal and entry into the bright light of the operating theater. We are pretty convinced that each of our bodies contains these objects along with others equally discrete and objective. And when it is time to renew our driver's license we feel that it is our moral duty to promise these removable things as gifts to needy strangers.

But the individual organs are scarcely known to us through ex-perience. I might feel that I know my heart by way of that cardiac thumping I feel in times of exertion (though surely my less percus-sive lungs are just as much at work). But, personally, I've always been a little vague on the location and activity of my kidneys. And the spleen? Gall bladder? Forget about it! Given that most of us live in a kind of carnal flow, living at best through what Deleuze and Guattari called "a body without organs," how is it that the body's anatomical organs have become so naturalized, so commonsensical, even so commodified, as self-evident *things* in today's world?[42]

Chinese doctors, contemplating biomedical knowledge, ask themselves questions like this. Though they incorporate little images of anatomical organs into some of their illustrations, for example, diagrams of the pathways used in acupuncture, TCM still seems to find the European anatomy tradition to be rather a bore.[43] The lungs, heart, or liver, positioned among the circulation tracks in acupuncture textbook illustrations, are sketched there more to orient the inexperienced reader and aid her imagination of the spatiality of the body than because they are an important component in the system being depicted. As I have argued elsewhere, TCM doctors tend to think of the anatomical structure as a relatively passive resultant—a deposit, as it were, like silt in a delta—of a constructive physiological process that demands to be understood on its own terms, not as product but as process. I made a similar argument some years ago in an article on female infertility, in which I suggested that a uterus becomes a salient thing for Chinese medicine only when a fetus is growing inside it.[44] The heart or kidney held in the hands or stashed in the Styrofoam cooler for transplant, the uterus removed in a hysterectomy—these may have a structural identity, but in the eyes of the Chinese doctor such an organ has lost its most important identifying features, its *functions* in a network of interacting things—dynamic *duixiang*—that sustain life.

Nevertheless, here's one of the delightful puzzles that presents itself to those of us who translate Chinese medicine: the Chinese medical classics, some of them dating back two thousand years, speak often of hearts, livers, kidneys, lungs, spleens and stomachs, urinary bladders, gall bladders, and intestines, large and small.[45] There is no doubt that the medical sages knew the contents of human bodies, and it is also clear that they—some of them, anyway—made reference to a "body *with* organs," Deleuze and Guattari notwithstanding—as a way of visualizing and working in bodily space. They located physiological activity as more or less inward, or more rising than falling, for example, making frequent reference to organs high or low, superficial or deep-seated.

But they and their modern heirs find the image of an organ depicted as an object floating in space, not as part of a system of living activity, useful only for the most primitive didactic demonstrations. An image of an internal organ might appear on a graphically engaging chart of physiological correlations, but these floating objects function more as mnemonics than as representations of a reality. Added to a chart like table 1, for example, images of hearts, livers, and lungs would work as icons and metonyms, not as pictures referring back to the object-body and the revelations of the dissection lab.[46]

How do TCM doctors think about those organs that are named in the classics, then? Modern Chinese medicine has a heavily theorized and systematized special field on this subject: visceral systems imagery, or *zangxiang xueshuo* (脏象学说). I want to conclude this chapter, then, with a consideration of the object nature of a "visceral system." This branch of knowledge in TCM offers profound resources for thinking about things, which I have been treating as the central question of ontology. And it opens to us, perhaps, a rather unusual kind of body or style of embodiment—perhaps in the end we can even imagine living a body with interpenetrating visceral systems of function (I am here using Sivin's full term), rather than discrete organs.[47] One could begin with mundane experience. It is not hard, for example, to notice the whole-body effects of a head or foot massage, a gut-wrenching image on television, a cotton swab in an itchy ear, or even a sudden sneeze. These flows of sensation can be well understood through the correlations of visceral systems activity.

Here's how, in *Knowing Practice*, I initially characterized Chinese medicine's organ-based visceral systems:

> Although the visceral systems are named with reference to an internal organ, they are not bounded or discrete sub-territories of an anatomically structured body. They are not, for example, livers that are homogeneously liver tissue from edge to edge, or hearts that can be removed and replaced with a mechanical organ that can be held in one hand. Rather they are interpenetrating systems of related functions that, nevertheless, have a definite spatial dimension. One can (indeed must) talk of up and down, in and out while describing Chinese visceral physiology; but Spleen and Liver visceral systems extend throughout the same bodily space with their differing domains of responsibility.[48]

This is a notion of the spatial organization of the human body that is both demanding and exciting. I recall explaining visceral systems to a colleague by comparison with the way late afternoon games were played when I lived at the College of Traditional Chinese Medicine in Guangzhou in the early 1980s: in the limited open space of one large playing field circled by a running track, too many students and faculty tried every day to play soccer, volleyball, and basketball, to jog, to lift weights, and to perform calisthenics in loudly counting groups. Watching all this energetic activity, I couldn't always figure out which individuals were playing soccer and which were playing volleyball; basketball players set up jump shots in the same parts of the field where soccer players dribbled toward an ad hoc goal marked by two bricks. I couldn't keep track of who was playing at what, but I was very impressed that the players themselves always seemed to know who was on their team and which of several balls was their object of interest. This image of interpenetrating but distinct games, organizing themselves around the movements of minimal and primitive but distinct objects, impressed my colleague mightily. A few years later, it was the only thing he remembered about my beloved research projects.

I don't want to push a sports field metaphor too far, but keep this booming and buzzing athletic field in mind as you consider table 1, which summarizes the domains belonging to each of the five master visceral systems. The table is oversimplified, but it captures something important about the visceral systems networks, understood as organic assemblages. This is evident as we read horizontally for each of the five systems: the heart (for example) rules blood, stores

Table 1. *Zang* Visceral Systems

Zang	Stores	Rules	Manifests in	Vents at
Heart	神 *shen*-spirit	blood, vessels	face	tongue
Lung	气 *qi*	clearing away, the watercourse	skin and body hair	nose
Spleen	津液 fluids	transmission and transformation, elevates clear fluids, blood flow, flesh, the four limbs	lips	mouth
Liver	血 blood	dredging and draining, dispersion upward and outward, sinews	nails	eyes
Kidney	精 *jing*-essence	accepts qi, fluids, marrow, bones	hair	ears genitals anus

shen-spirit, unfolds in the vessels, manifests in the face, and vents at the tongue. Not shown in the table is the fact that the heart visceral system is affiliated to a parallel "hollow organ," that of the small intestine system, and the fact that heart system functions are facilitated by flow in the Hand Lesser Yin Heart Meridian (or circulation track).[49]

To see how the interpenetrating playing fields metaphor applies, compare the heart system with the liver system. Liver rules processes of dredging and draining as well as dispersion (of qi) upward and outward; it stores blood, unfolds in the sinews, vents at the eyes, and manifests in the nails; it is affiliated to the gall bladder system and unfolds in the Foot Reverting Yin Liver Meridian. While the heart rules the vessels, the liver rules the sinews. But these two reticular networks, vessels and sinews, are intertwined throughout the body and even intimately dependent on each other—how can they be seen as aspects of two separate things, a heart and a liver? Moreover, what is the difference in practice between "ruling blood" (the heart) and "storing blood" (the liver)?

Let's address such questions by reflecting on one key verb. As a translator of Chinese medicine into English, I have always been intrigued and challenged by the forms of activity that are of interest to the clinician. What English verbs can I use that will not distort these processes, which I and my students are not very accustomed to speaking about? What does it mean, physiologically, to say that the heart *rules* blood (*xin zhu xue* 心主血) or that the liver "rules" dredging and draining (*gan zhu shuxie* 肝主疏泄)? Well, to understand this verb, *zhu*, or "rules," I'm afraid we have to steep ourselves not only in clinical experience but also in classical ideas about rulership, a topic on which ancient Chinese philosophy focused much attention for several hundred years in the Warring States, Qin, and Han Periods. The original medical writing on visceral systems dates from that classic era, after all, and we might suspect that the proto-medical theorists writing in the classic age were thinking about the practice of power relations in wider worlds as they wrote (see appendix 2).

Indeed, when we note (as many have) the liberal use of words involving governance in the most technical ancient medical writing, it seems clear that these healers and thinkers were composing a body that could serve as the ontological foundation of an antique state—a polity that was, at the time, violently under construction. A human body envisioned as interpenetrating networks that channeled powers throughout a decentered system might be read as natural proof that rule of any kind, at any scale, could not be totalitarian, nor could it extend its reach only over discretely bounded territories. Rule over territory and people, rule over vital energies—both, for Chinese antiquity, were a matter of condensed nodes (like organs, like capital cities) anchoring unbounded networks of lively activity or emanating influence, a matter of gatherings and scatterings of qi and of people.

So when a Chinese doctor explains to a student or intern that the heart rules *shen*-spirit while the liver rules blood, he is evoking a particular theory of power and responsibility. This form of power has been sustained and elaborated throughout the history of medicine in China, even though in the domain of government it has been rather completely transformed with the rise of the modern Chinese nation-state. *Zhu* "rule" is not the total domination of a power-holder over his weak and passive subjects; rather, *zhu*—even in today's TCM—looks more like ruling through non-action (*wuwei* 无为), ruling as an exemplar, anchoring social order as an unmoved mover, or providing a source of virtue and power (*de* 德) in the social world.[50] When ruling by non-action is refracted through medicine, in the heart system, for example, we no longer see a pumping organ that pushes blood through a fixed network of vessels. The force that makes blood flow is the qi-energy intrinsic to blood as it sponta-neously circulates through living bodies. It is, in other words, the qi-blood relationship that is "making fluid move" through the body. This is a very decentered forcefulness that could not be sustained by a merely mechanical pump. Those things that are ruled in various sites of the body (the spreading network of vessels, in the case of the heart) are already active. They don't need to be set in motion; perhaps, rather, when therapy is at issue, they need to be guided, nudged, or redirected in their flow.

Conclusion

Given the subtleties we find in the verbs of physiology, and given the dispersed and interpenetrating character of the five great organ systems, what are the commonsense things belonging to the body? Does the work of qi in our embodied experiences feel right some-how, whether or not we have been reached by acupuncture needles? What is the reality of the entities—diseases or patterns—that (with-out doubt) are forms of affliction in the body and its systems? In-deed, can *the body* itself be a commonplace, universal sort of thing in a world that accommodates many modes of doing "medicine"?[51] With these questions we land in a space beyond cultural difference, beyond linguistic translation, and beyond the merely conceptual.

Medicines of all kinds work with real stuff. The pattern of dis-order that is a thing for Lu Guangxin and his whole generation (at least) of Chinese medicine doctors; the heart, lungs, spleen, liver, and kidneys that together and inseparably fill the body with activity; the minimal substances that flow in this body (*shen*-spirit, blood, qi, fluids, and *jing*-essence)—these are not just cultural or imaginary things belonging to a world that has receded from view or, worse, perished under the weight of its ontological errors. Rather, to para-phrase W. I. Thomas, the Chicago sociologist, situations—and what is a thing if not a contingent situation?—defined as real are real in their consequences. These things are experienced, known, and used in clinics, classrooms, workshops, and kitchens throughout the world.[52] Yet the things addressed in a different language world are still difficult to recognize in the frame of a modernist metaphysics. Chinese medicine, with its simplest, most commonly encountered, and most taken-for-granted objects, bespeaks the plural and rela-tional universe in which pragmatists like William James and meta-physicians like Zhang Zai have invited us to try to live.

In the next two lectures I will consider how it is possible to think and act in a universe where so many of the objects present at hand for the Chinese doctor are ever under construction, always becom-ing, expressing their propensities quirkily under particular historical conditions, but no less real for all that.[53]

3

Thought: Knowing in Practice

医者意也
yizhe yi ye
Medicine is thought.[1]

In the last chapter I observed that "diagnosis" in biomedicine refers to a way of knowing apart, or making things like diseases discrete, like objects. Chinese medical doctors, by contrast, resist the cutting action, the knowing apart, of diagnosis. They believe their ways of knowing are able not only to recognize living things *as* things but to understand them in process, with both knower and known fully entangled in active vital networks. In constructivist mode, I spoke of medical things—diseases and patterns, organs and visceral systems—as being composed and assembled even as they are being perceived or discovered. To know life's processes without dissecting the dead, to understand a body's events without controlling variables in a laboratory or disciplining factors in a clinical trial, this requires a kind of educated perception that is not only or exclusively Chinese. The knowing gaze, bodily engagement, and thoughtful analysis of the medical practitioner are preeminently practical and clinical, and probably typical of medical work everywhere and everywhen.

Yet it is much more common in the writings of Chinese medical doctors than it is in biomedical discourses to refer to the "thoughtful" dimension of clinical work. (See appendix 2 for an extended and fascinating example.) In modern biomedical contexts, "thought" and "the clinical" do not often appear together as themes in authoritative discourse. To some, "clinical thought" might seem as awkward a combination as that old joke: military intelligence, an oxymoron. Our epigraph, "Medicine is thought," however, challenges the modern idea that medicine belongs more to the technical sciences than to the interpretive humanities. What would clinical/medical thought look like?

This chapter cannot promise a philosophy of the mind or even an intellectual history of Chinese medical thought. What we think of as "thought" is so various: its diversities are rich, its ambitions are wild, its speculations are creative, and, above all, its relationship to multiple and changing languages is so very intimate. William James challenged the modern rationalist divide between thing and thought and treated thinking as a practice; anthropologists explore the thought of nonhumans to discover ontological pluralism; biologists find mind in whales and octopuses.[2] I will suggest below that thought for Chinese healers might be inseparable from general patterns of cosmic emergence. Is thought nothing other than an aspect—one of many—of the ceaseless birth and transformation of the myriad things? I'd like to think so, but an anthropologist cannot presume to decide the nature of thought, even when she confines herself to one historical moment (the 1980s to the present) in one geographical and cultural location (the Chinese medical profession). This anthropologist is fairly certain that she cannot accurately represent the "thought process" of even her closest associates who work as clinicians, even after much conversation. In this chapter, instead, I hope to keep the field I am calling "thought" open to question, attentive to creative action, and appreciative of philosophical writing in Chinese about medicine and the work of treating bodily disorders. Rather than summarize TCM thought (this would be far too daunting given the size and diversity of the literature!), I here discuss a few examples of how some Chinese healers think about, represent, and practically express their work of thinking.

But first it must be pointed out, Chinese medicine is not the only form of medicine that thinks in the clinic while encountering the complexities of a living person and being required, urgently, to act. Far from it. I paraphrased Nathan Sivin in chapter 1, in his assertion that medicine everywhere is more an art than a science. This is a rather scandalous assertion in a Chinese climate that has been utterly committed, since the early twentieth century, to scientific modernity. Modern TCM, being required in the mid-twentieth century to construct a national education and training system that could produce good "traditional medicine" doctors, has had no choice but to think, reflexively and abstractly, about how the art and science of clinical thought should be structured, cultivated, and flexibly and responsibly practiced. "Western medical" practitioners in China have not been put in a similar defensive position; they tend to believe that they are operating, in their clinics, with a system of techniques deriving directly from scientific facts that were established mostly in the West.[3]

We can learn much from Chinese medicine's modern pedagogical strategies and philosophical reflexivity. Historical and cultural scholarship in China on "traditional medicines" has been fortunate: twentieth-century leaders in the development of TCM have been not only scientists and clinicians, they have also been teachers and philosophers. And they have written a lot about their practice and their thought. These writers often speak of a TCM "style of thought" (*siwei fangshi* 思维方式), their usage implicitly invoking all manner of multiplicities in reasoning and imagining. The metaphysical visions of "the ancients" are almost inaccessible to those schooled in more recent styles of thought. What was thought for a Neo-Confucian like Zhang Zai (author of the chapter 2 epigraph)? For objectivists like TCM's 1920s critics? For investigators designing randomized-controlled clinical trials? In the world of TCM, thinking people (like, for example, Zhang Dong, see appendix 2, and Liao Yuqun, this chapter's footnote 1) still read speculative philosophy from several thousand years ago in search of novel styles of thought and clinical guidance. In this chapter I will translate from their discourse, their world, and their practices of not only thinking but also teaching and healing.

Gathering Patterns as Clinical Thought

In the last chapter, I introduced a widely accepted modern approach to the logic of the clinical encounter known as *bianzheng lunzhi,* discerning pattern and determining therapy (schematized in figure 1). One of my aims in chapter 2 was to demonstrate the gathered character of the *zhenghou,* that contingent clinical thing, a pattern of disorder. Rising along the left side of the diagram in figure 1 are some disciplined methods, or forms of analytical reasoning (the term is *bianzheng fangfa* 辨证方法), that have characterized the practice of many TCM doctors trained since the 1960s. In the diagram, some of these methods of discerning are conventionally named: eight rubrics, illness factors, visceral systems, and so on. For those practitioners who are uncomfortable with the epistemological cutting involved in the knowing apart that diagnoses ontological disease, *bianzheng lunzhi* offers what might be called cognosis, or knowledge through recognition of a pattern that is coming together: knowing together, we could say. Or even, gathering.[4]

But the verbs that could be used in writing in English about this mode of clinical thought have often given me pause. After all, thought is so many kinds of activity. The translator of the *bianzheng lunzhi* process is not helped by knowing exactly what is observable in practice: no one verb can capture the character of the mental activity required to discern a pattern of disorder.[5] Is this clinical thought a work of analyzing, assembling, classifying, recollecting, modeling, interrogating, explaining, understanding, contextualizing, tracing, connecting, correlating, knowing . . . ? Even the textbook list of standard analytic methods (eight rubrics, illness factors, etc.) is rather miscellaneous; these methods do not add up to one big methodology of thinking, and they are quite capable of giving contradictory results when (as is usual) they are used together.

Before we draw closer to the pattern-discerning process, however, and while reflecting on the ambiguity and openness of the thought process in the clinical encounter, let's not forget that we're talking about thought and reasoning in general. Consider, for example, the verb in the epigraph, "Medicine is thought."[6] This is an ancient phrase that has recently been often invoked by those in China who build on (or forge afresh) the philosophical and theoretical foundations for medical things, thought, and action. The verbal form in *yizhe yi ye* is the most basic copula of classical Chinese, the syntactical "*ye*" that characterizes and defines a thing by pointing at another thing, making an equivalence. *Yizhe yi ye* has an emphatic quality, a tone of voice that clears away the cobwebs and states the obvious fact, which we might be in danger of missing: "Medicine really, after all, is nothing but thinking!"[7] And this copula works both ways, logically. Thought is also medical healing, or at least among the varieties of thought "medicine" is an important sort. That is to say, the realm of thought includes medicine, so medicine is always more than a mechanical technology of modifying well-understood pathologies. *Yizhe yi ye* thus beautifully charters the task of this chapter: to persuade you that any thinking person should want to grasp how Chinese medicine, in particular, thinks.

But be warned! Much of this chapter explicates rather technical methods in modern systematic TCM. Even though I have (over) simplified them, these practices and concepts, these unfamiliar things, are not easy for most of us to follow. The figures and tables are intended to help, and there will be some redundancies as I return frequently to philosophical fundamentals. But it might also be wise for some readers to simply skip the clinical technicalities and look for the scattered philosophical nuggets among the detailed methods.

Patterning and Disciplining, Formulas and Medicines (*Li Fa Fang Yao* 理法方药)

In 1935, an influential historian, publisher, and medical practitioner named Xie Guan wrote a lapidary history and explication of traditional Chinese medicine, *Sources and Currents of Chinese Medicine*. It's a small book, written in concise and resonant classical Chinese, and it was influential for a while, though it never achieved the fame I think it deserves.[8] At the time Xie was writing, his field was in crisis, with medical practitioners throughout China having narrowly escaped an attempted national ban on their work at the hands of modernizing biomedical interests.[9] China was already at war with Japan, and the nation was also deeply divided by warlordism and the struggle between the Nationalist and Communist Parties. The proponents of what was then called "National Medicine" (*guoyi* 国医) had little time and few resources to advance the modernizing and conserving—and also nationalist—agenda that many of them shared. Heightened politics notwithstanding, Xie Guan accomplished much as a scholar and a theorist. He also liked to insist that "medicine is thought."

Another of his pithy slogans is frequently cited in Chinese medicine today: *li fa fang yao* (理法方药), or patterns, disciplines, formulas, medicines. (See box 2, where a four-term model following Xie Guan can be contrasted with the now more hegemonic *bianzheng lunzhi* model diagrammed in figure 1.) It was often asserted to me when I was first studying Chinese medicine in Guangzhou that these four words *li fa fang yao* "epitomize the essence of the field." I didn't understand this at all at the time—my awkward translation here indicates how miscellaneous and inadequate this phrase appeared to me; it did not seem to be a coherent list of parallel things, nor did it sum up an essence of any kind, as far as I could see. (But let's stick with the awkward translation of "patterns, disciplines, formulas, medicines" for the time being.)

Lately I've been reflecting on these words, after finally reading Xie Guan's intellectual history in which he proposed this slogan. Let's look especially at the first component of his four-term list: *li* 理 is a term of vast importance in the history of Chinese philosophy, especially thanks to the Neo-Confucian movement of the Song and Ming Periods. Though its most primitive meaning is "pattern"—as in the grain of wood or the current of a stream—it has long been translated by anglophone philosophers, especially those steeped in Zhu Xi's Neo-Confucian ethics and metaphysics, as "principle." But that translation arguably over-idealizes the concept, even as it was

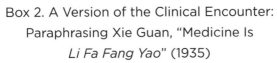

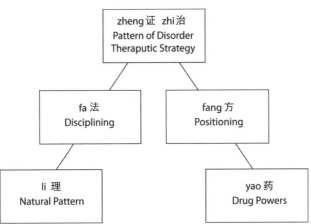

Figure 2. "Medicine is li, fa, fang, yao*"*

Figure 2 presents a sequence of events: Natural Pattern—Disciplining—Pattern of Disorder/Therapeutic Strategy—Positioning—Drug Powers.

Rising through the left side, the clinician *gathers* manifestations (signs arising as *li*) and correlates them with invisible processes in a variety of disciplined ways using a few "traditional" analytic methods (*fa*). Descending through the right side, s/he *assembles* a customized therapeutic intervention positioning (*fang*) the powers of materia medica drawn from nature (*yao*) into relation with each other in a drug formula. The top of the order is occupied by the pattern of disorder (*zhenghou*), a temporary and contingent thing expressed as a condition requiring intervention, and by the therapeutic strategy (*zhifa*) that guides the choice of drugs and their proportional positioning in the formula.

continued

Let me restate this sequence using details from a case of high fever, which I discussed at greater length in *Knowing Practice* (see especially pp. 47–50):

The presenting signs, *li* manifestations of pathological process, were high fever; agitation and irritability; dry mouth and excessive thirst; red face and foul mouth odor; tongue and lips dry and parched; delirious speech; no appetite; constipation; pulse smooth and accelerated; and tongue coating yellow, thick, dry.

The methods of disciplined correlation, or *fa,* used in this case appear to have been (at least) an analysis of the listed signs according to an eight rubrics classification method and read through a four sectors dynamics. These analytics were supplemented by certain ideas drawn from illness factor analysis. All of these methods (*bianzhengfa* 辨证法) are ways to make pathological-processual sense of the long list of diverse manifestations that emerged and presented as *li,* or pathological signs. These methods, in other words, enabled a disciplined gathering of an increasingly coherent condition.

This gathering culminated in a *zheng*, or the *zhenghou* (see the discussion of Lu Guangxin's usage in chapter 2), which was named as "spring warm repletion in the yang visceral systems." And then *zhi,* or *zhifa* (治法), a treatment principle or plan, could be explicitly named as well: "clear above and drain below."

Because drugs are known to have powers—in this case, clearing and draining powers—and because they can target specific visceral systems which do their work relatively high or low in the body, the *fang* was designed with these powers and tendencies in mind. In this case the doctor drew on several classic formulas, Barrier Cooling Powder and Ginseng–White Tiger Decoction, modifying them to address some of the specific signs and symptoms at issue. The technical considerations he had to keep in mind as he adopted and reassembled these formulas are sometimes referred to as *chufang* 处方, or "the positioning of a formula."

And then there are the drugs, *yao*, themselves. This case of Spring Warm was treated with formulas heavily reliant on fresh gypsum and rehmannia rhizome, but each of the three prescriptions used contained eleven drugs, carefully quantified to occupy the right "positions" of power relative to each other within the formula. And, of course, each of the three formulas changed as the symptomatic manifestations of pathological process changed.

Out of loyalty to Xie Guan's brilliant and influential slogan, "medicine is *li fa fang yao*," I should point out that many don't feel that the top box is necessary and suggest that the *zheng* pattern of disorder (or pattern of disharmony, as Kaptchuk would have it) is a relatively modern invention that is meant to compare with, and contrast with, the biomedical concept of ontological disease.[a] Xie Guan's formula, still much quoted in professional TCM circles, fails to mention *zheng* and *zhi,* perhaps because at the time he was writing they were not thematized at the center of TCM logic. Indeed there is much evidence in the contemporary and canonical literature of TCM that the art of "positioning" a drug formula is much more highly valued, even in contemporary practice, than some well-schooled ability to properly discern and name a pattern.[b] And plenty of clinicians find it rather pointless and burdensome to have to articulate a "treatment principle" when they already have in mind a properly positioned formula, classical or invented on the spot. The therapeutic assemblage achieved through the right-hand side of this diagrammed encounter might be best thought of as a practical harnessing of the ever-emergent powers of natural things—such as plants.[c] And, looking backward to when the suffering patient entered the consulting room, the manifestations or signs of disorder that Xie Guan called *li*—a complex keyword if ever there was one in the Chinese philosophical tradition—is an arrival in the clinic of a not-yet-tamed multiplicity of natural (if pathological) instances of becoming.

continued

One last thought on this cryptic diagram: the events of the clinical encounter do not just divide between right and left, gathering and assembling, disciplining and positioning. The "bottom half" has a special importance as it is constantly gathered up into the "top half." The yang repletion that became visible through *fa* disciplining methods has not exited the world of spontaneous natural becoming that is *li*. It is, perhaps, just a more refined form of natural pattern, given that the doctor and his thinking cannot stand outside of *li*. And the formulas that combine the powers of natural drugs do not purify or refine those drugs into a set of, for example, "active ingredients." The plants and minerals, the rehmannia and gypsum in this case, that are assembled according to formula in the pharmacy rooms of the clinic are important agents in this actor-networked sequence of events throughout the whole process. And each drug retains its own naturally complex character. Should *li* and *yao* be seen as foundational to the *li fa fang yao* process that is medicine? Chinese doctors act as if they see things that way.

a. Kaptchuk, *Web That Has No Weaver*.

b. See, e.g., Zhang, *Original Qi, Vital Machine* and clinical logic through cases. But also note that the corpus of works on formulary is huge and perhaps the most frequently consulted type of literature in the broad field of TCM.

c. The trope of assemblage has become very important in post-colonial science studies; see, e.g., Verran, "On Assemblage."

used by the most metaphysical of Chinese philosophers.[10] A principle, after all, can be drawn apart from the things it is believed to inform; it claims a rather wispy and ideal existence that only gains weightiness when it is reunified with its material expression. Medical uses of "*li*," then—never not weighty—would perhaps prefer it be glossed as (bodily) "pattern" rather than (mental) "principle."

One way to grasp what Xie Guan and my Guangzhou teachers might have been thinking when they recommended that I reflect on *li* and its three following terms is to look at modern dictionary definitions. Here are some short glosses provided in a very standard dictionary, along with some comments in italics:[11] *Li* is (1) streaks in material structures, wood grain [*A very concrete and individual pattern, right? Not a free-standing object or idealizable principle.*]; (2) principle, reason, logic [*Is this the idealism of "principle" as an element in reasoning?*]; (3) among the natural sciences, physics [*The science of natural dynamic patterns?*]; (4) manage, control, cope with [*As a supervisor would manage the work of employees.*]; (5) edit, order, sort out [*This is very mundane, I must put my affairs in order, organize the bookcases.*]; (6) express a negative opinion on someone else's verbal behavior [*This last recalls a common oral negative:* "buli wo, *don't mind me (I'm just a bystander).*"].

If *li* is all these philosophical and mundane things at once, and if it is used as a verbal (which is pretty clear in the slogan *li fa fang yao*), then it helps us quite a bit as we try to think Chinese medical thinking. Let's provisionally gloss it, in the context of *li fa fang yao*, as "noticing and ordering things through attending to their natural patterns."

The four-character slogan *li fa fang yao* helped Xie Guan and his intellectual descendants make a case for TCM as they tried to modernize and systematize their field. Note again the structure of the phrase: it might be parsed as a verb and a result, then another verb and result. Two predicates with medicine as the implicit subject of both. If pattern is a form of reasoning, then what Chinese medicine does, Xie was saying, is *reason* (*li*) its way to a discipline or method (*fa*), and having arrived at that method it can compose a drug *formula* (that is, formulate a prescription, *fang*); only then can it properly assemble the bundle of concrete *medicines* (*yao*) that will be handed over to the patient.[12] I will return to the work of composing drugs together in *fang* formulas in chapter 4; and the last term, *yao,* or "medicines," reminds us of the question of the actively gathered *thing* that I considered in chapter 2.

But of the four words in Xie Guan's important formula, *li* is the most powerful notion. By the twentieth century, modernist ideas about reason, logic, truth, and science ruled in China (recall the dictionary list!). By adopting for Chinese medicine a philosophical term that encompassed modern science, reason, and truth, while dragging along with it a long history and a vast literature in Chinese (which literature partly retained the term's primary meaning as pattern), Xie Guan was being very canny. When we reflect on and read about the historical moment in which Xie Guan was writing, it appears that he was making an early gesture in the invention of a scientistic theory-practice divide for China.

He was not alone. The political pressures that were making "theory" into a stratum of discourse underpinning an ancient clinical art are too complex to describe here.[13] But some policy makers at the time were arguing for keeping the effective herbal drugs of Chinese medicine and discarding everything else, especially the "traditional thinking" of the field. It is not an accident, then, that Xie Guan's *li fa fang yao* took hold among TCM advocates in the 1930s and was still urged on me as an important guide for Chinese medical development fifty years after Xie first voiced the formula. He and his contemporaries realized, as their nation struggled toward modern statehood, a modern science must have "theoretical foundations," it must be "rational." But a self-consciously traditional and national medicine must find its rational foundation in something homegrown, and classical East Asian philosophy offered no shortage of resources for systematic thought (see appendix 2). With formulas like *li fa fang yao*, the field both resisted scientism and exemplified a broader vision of science as secular reason.

There is an immensely complex stance and practice involved in the way that "patterning" (*li*) is thought to produce a method (*fa*, a specific form of intervention in illness), and this stance is repeated, as the composition of the formula (*fang*) yields a structured collection of things (*yao*), which is to say, a bundle of loose drugs, medicines you can take home and boil up into a soup (*tang* 汤). Theory-practice, theory-practice, a science both ancient and modern declares itself in this phrase. And *li,* or the grain and pattern of becoming, rules in the field of medicine.

Manifest Signs and the Four Examinations

Having promised some empirical answers to how medical reasoning might work, let's focus now on the "discerning patterns" side of the diagram in figure 1, beginning with the four examinations. The importance of this step in the process was reinforced for me when I accompanied a group of American students to visit a Chinese medical clinic in 2017. Our group was lucky to be hosted by a senior doctor who, with a very tolerant patient by his side, gave a brief lecture introducing the field of Chinese medicine. What Dr. Ping most wanted to emphasize—in the context of this self-consciously "traditional" private clinic—was the four methods of examination, which is to say, the perceptual phase of the clinical encounter. He proceeded to demonstrate by performing these examination methods on the patient: looking at the tongue, palpating the pulse, drawing our attention to facial color, rehearsing a bit of the patient's history (box 3). Like so many other experts I have spoken with over the years, he

Box 3. The Four Methods of Examination

Looking Examination: general vitality and vigor; facial color; color of tongue body, quality of tongue coating, tongue shape; body gesture and disposition.

Listening/Smelling Examination: speech, breathing, coughing, voice quality; unusual odors.

Asking Examination: illness onset, experienced symptoms, attitudes, worries; family history of illness. Fevers, perspiration, aches and pains, internal feelings of pressure, excreta, diet and appetite, thirst, menses, discharge, sleep patterns.

Palpating Examination: pulse (three sites at each level, shallow, middle, deep, on both wrists), twenty-eight possible pulse images can be felt. Also, palpation of sites of pain, abdominal fullness or yieldingness, discomfort with or without palpation.

obviously considered the disciplined perception enabled by the four examinations to be the foundation of Chinese medical thinking.[14]

Dr. Ping was showing us a widely taught, even required protocol for clinical work in traditional medicine. But, we could ask, why were the many ways in which doctors read and learn from patients' bodies organized into *the* four examinations, and, further, made into a protocol religiously taught to medical students? We could also ask, why are there only four? Do the four examinations as taught (and lectured to us in that clinic in 2017) really reflect the subtleties and multiplicities of a good doctor's perception? In practice, these four modes of clinical observation tend to *limit* the infinite information that can be gleaned from a sufferer's body and history. After all, from a patient's point of view, a human body is rather what William James called a quasi-chaos.[15] James figures this quasi-chaos as a kind of unknowable physical core around which floats a "vast cloud of experiences," only some of which can become part of the perceptual experience of another, in this case, a diagnostician.

Limits are essential in a medical encounter, as I reluctantly recognize every time I talk to my doctor, and then leave her clinic a little uncertain whether she has heard and understood all aspects of my condition (or, even cares to "understand"). Her version and mine of what counts as symptomatic differ somewhat; I present her with a quasi-chaos, and she cuts down my inarticulate messiness to information that can usefully inform her diagnosis. Some of our experiences as patients are worth no medical attention, whereas other symptomatic conditions—which might not be conscious experiences at all—must be tricked into showing themselves, for example with blood tests, ultrasound, sphygmometers, and other equipment.

The four examinations impose a discipline, then, but they also collect quite a lot of information. As can be seen in the lists in box 3, these methods are looking, listening/smelling, asking, and palpating. Clearly, this is a protocol that is attentive to a great deal of patient and doctor experience—colors of tongue range from carmine to nearly black, with tongue coating that can have not only different colors but qualities like dryness, thickness, greasiness, patchiness, and so on; there are twenty-eight possible pulse qualities discernable at eighteen possible sites on the wrists;[16] there are differential breathing sounds and weird voice effects to be listened to; and then there are the reported qualities of urine and stool, sleeping patterns, experiences of appetite and indigestion, grumpiness or euphoria, excessive dreams, and so on. The results of the four examinations are more than lists of symptoms; rather they amount to a phenomenology of pathological process in the experience of both patient and doctor. They collect aspects of the patient's experiences of disorder, expertly perceiving and discriminating qualities perceptible on the surface of a life in a kind of radical empiricist mode of attention. The signs of illness are expressions of a natural pathological process—they are surface manifestations whose generative sources are nonvisible interior processes.

But studying the lists in box 3, you might protest! Your primary care physician in New Haven or Chicago, or a medical student studying physical examination and history taking, would quickly point out that this method fails to catch many important things. Exact readings of blood pressure and body temperature are missing, neither the heartbeat nor the optic fundus nor the cervix is examined, neurological reflexes are not tested, and of course every structure that would be visualized with X-rays, CT scanning, and MRI remains in the dark. This last figure of speech—and real situation—helps us to see something important about that dark space of the body interior from which the manifest disorder rises to the surface. The four examinations collect *surface manifestations* almost exclusively, especially if we consider that the patient's verbal account of his symptomatic experience is yet another kind of manifestation, made present in speech in the space of the clinic for the consideration of the doctor.[17]

Modern Chinese medicine has only partly adopted the visualizing technologies that help biomedicine detect our body's silent lesions—the tumor, the malformed optic nerve, the colonic polyp—and this neglect of technology is often seen as a failure and a shortcoming of the field. But Chinese medical polemicists point out in parallel that biomedicine lacks phenomenological sophistication. Both its vision-centered modes of perception and its whole-body systematics are weak: so-called Western medicine is deaf to the many qualities resonating through the wrist pulses, and disorders of the whole body—metabolic or immune system disease, for example—have to be thought about and managed piecemeal—at best with drug cocktails—rather than treated "rationally," as a processual *li* "pattern."

How do the four examinations fit into Chinese medical knowing practice? What role do they play in a reasoning process? What part of *li fa fang yao* are they? It is easy to see them as a kind of medical semiotics, which is to say, a disciplined way of reading signs. Reading for meaning, we might even say. We are all familiar with this form of reading, whether or not we are physicians. Suffering from a bad cough, lower back pain, migraines, forgetfulness, we put together a narrative that explains why this set of symptoms (there are always several) has happened now, together, to me and not to my relatives or friends. And we extend this narrative to predict, hopefully, how long it will take for our symptomatic discomforts to change or go away.

But the stories we tell ourselves as patients and sufferers are idiosyncratic and unreliable compared to those that are developed in the pattern-discerning process. The four examinations are a reasoned protocol that yields information that Chinese doctors can think with; understood as indexes of pathological processes affecting the whole body, the set of signs a practitioner collects is placed in relation to the knowledge accumulated in China's much-vaunted "2000 years of medical experience" in ways to which we will soon turn. If I am told that I suffer from "deficient spleen function with damp heat"—as I have been, actually, and as Dr. Ping's patient was also told when we visited that clinic in August 2017—I might still feel that my Chinese doctor has failed to see the whole picture of my personal afflictions.[18] But given that the pattern the doctor discerns can yield a carefully crafted intervention, that is, a "formula" and "medicines" tailored to the state of pathophysiological play in my body, which he has inferred in a skilled reading, I have to be impressed with the sensitivity of his account to my body and its meanings.

But let me approach this emphasis on the four examinations, the discerning process, and the knowing practice of which they are a part in a slightly more historical way. Here are some lines from an absolutely classic 1959 book called *Introduction to Chinese Medicine*.[19] These remarks are from the preface written by the author Qin Bowei, an important founder of modern Chinese medicine:

> The Chinese Communist Party has long emphasized our nation's medical heritage, telling us: Chinese medicine and pharmacy is a great treasure-house.[20] . . . When Chinese medicine treats disease, it centrally relies on an integrated set of therapeutic methods consisting of patterning and disciplining, formulating and medicines [*li fa fang yao*]. I recognize the surface appearances (面貌 *mianmao*) of Chinese medicine from these four aspects. Through them we can understand Chinese medicine's specificity and grasp Chinese medicine's regular patterns of treating illness, and thus adopt the most correct approach to learning Chinese medicine. So in this book's account the various topics are divided up under the four sections of theory (*lilun*), methodology (*faze*), formulary (*fangji*), and pharmaceuticals (*yaowu*) so as to give a more detailed introduction. [These terms are a version of *li fa fang yao*.]

This is just one of many possible examples where Xie Guan's pithy formula of *li fa fang yao* is recapitulated (prominently and under the aegis of the People's Republic of China's Ministry of Health) long after the 1930s, just as it was repeated to me by my authoritative teachers in a 1980s Chinese medical college. It is interesting that Xie's *li* of the 1930s has by 1959 been transformed into the modern term for theory, *lilun*.[21]

But what is really impressive about this quotation from Qin's preface, for present purposes, is his mention of surface appearances. The word he used for this, *mianmao*, is not a medical word, and as far as I know hardly anyone later picked up this notion of "recognizing surface appearances" for their writing about the four examinations or any other component of the pattern-discerning and therapy-determining process. Perhaps the *reading* process characteristic of medical semiotics was already so firmly established as a method of reasoning that no particular comment was required—this would also be the case for Western medicine, by the way. But look at the logic of this statement. Perhaps like Dr. Ping in the clinic I visited in 2017, Dr. Qin is here putting his "recognition" of appearances at the foundation of his thinking practice: as clinician, he processes what appears on the surface through pattern, method, formula, and even drugs to deal with the (even more defining) task of reading signs. In the process, this becomes knowing from experience. The disciplined four examinations are the beginning of discernment; their signs present themselves to be read on the surfaces of bodies and in patient's accounts of illness experience.

Manifest Images and Their Sources

In these pages we have seen Qin Bowei's "surface appearances" before, and the word we have used for them, *xiang,* has often been translated as "image." The four examinations lists in box 3 includes some "images": pulse image and tongue image are very important, as Dr. Ping emphasized. With regard to visceral systems imagery, mentioned in chapter 2, "*xiang*" is a visible image that makes visceral activity apparent. Examples might be a flush in the face, where the heart system "manifests," or bloodshot eyes, where the liver system "vents." The name for this way of thinking, visceral systems imagery, presumes that the hidden activity of the visceral systems networks throws up an image that can be perceived by the senses of an attentive observer.

The most thoughtful (and witty) usage of the word *xiang* was discussed in chapter 2, when I talked about Lu Guangxin's word for object or thing, which was *duixiang* 对象, or the image we face. This last notion is suggestive for our efforts to understand ways of thinking (and reading, and translating, and even intervening). Why? Because—and here I must dip once again into metaphysics, à la Lu Guangxin—the active cosmos *throws up* the appearances that face us. These *duixiang* are, of course, *things*, myriad and intertransforming, as are we.[22] It is not just *images* or manifestations we need to apprehend and relate to each other if we are to intervene in illness; we need to grasp the *process* by which they are generated, get a feel for and even participate in that more whole and unitary Way that brings the life of bodies into existence.

Chinese medicine holds that pathological and physiological processes of the whole body are more unitary and more coherent—more holistic, the modern theorists say—than the miscellany of "myriad" phenomena—for example, illness signs—that present themselves to our human senses. The endless transformative life process has its patterns, its regularities, its grain or current, but it is also one Dao and can be grasped as a kind of inexhaustible unity by the skilled doctor. (Modern author Liao Yuqun says, "[This Way is] graspable in thought, but it is hard to transmit in words" [可以意会，难于言传].[23]

Put another way, medical semiotics, the reading of manifest signs, is not just a historically standardized way of putting symptoms into the form of a pattern, one that is visible to an "outside" observer and could be "transmitted in words." Rather, clinical thought is, for many TCM practitioners, an entire metaphysics, a mode of thought that can begin to see, feel, and work with some ultimate sources.[24] But to see how such ultimates might be graspable, we must start at the manifest and myriad "end" of the path of becoming, or the Way.

The reading, interpreting, classifying, and making actionable of the signs or *xiang* of illness is a practical problem, one that often faces the clinician in the quasi-chaos of a particular human life. Each of us is an unstable and contingent gathering among the myriad things. Medical people often refer to unceasing genesis and transformation, the *shengsheng huahua* (生生化化) of the manifest things of nature as they try to stay on top of the microevolutions of illness and cure.[25] There is a paragraph from the *Zhuangzi* (c. fourth century BCE) that in its delightful teeming confusion well expresses the *shengsheng huahua* of the myriad things of perception:

> The sorts of the myriad things are the work of the most minute seeds. In the water the seeds become Break Vine, but on the shore they become Frog's Robe. If they grow on the hillside they become Hill Slippers; if Hill Slippers find good soil they become Crowsfoot. The roots of Crowsfoot turn into maggots and their leaves turn into butterflies. Soon the butterflies transform and turn into those insects that hatch under the stove: they look like snakes, taking the form of nymphs in molt, and then they are called *Quduo*. After a thousand days, *Quduo* become birds, those known as Dry Left-over Bones Birds. The spit of Left-over Bones Birds

becomes *Simi* bugs; *Simi* are those bugs that eat wine dregs. *Yilu* bugs are born from those wine-eaters, *Huangkuang* bugs are born from *Jiuyou* bugs, and *Maorui* bugs are born from Rot Grubs. Sheep's Groom grass couples with the old bamboo that for a long time has put out no fresh shoots, and this coupling gives birth to Green Serenity bugs. Serenity bugs give birth to leopards, leopards give birth to horses, horses give birth to humans; humans return to the unfathomable works. The ten thousand things all come out of the works, and all return to the works.[26]

All those untranslated words for (possibly) bugs are not more meaningful to contemporary Chinese scholars than they are to us, reading Zhuangzi in English. But the fluidity of being and the pervasiveness of becoming are utterly clear in this passage from chapter 18, "Arriving at Happiness" (*zhile* 至乐).

Zhang Dong, author of the preface excerpted in appendix 2, draws on this same passage from the *Zhuangzi* to emphasize not the myriad phenomena encountered as a miscellany in his medical practice, but the way in which human life—apparently emergent from leopards and horses only about five minutes ago!—"comes out of the works and returns to the works."[27] In his preface, he begins to explain the logic of his own clinical efforts to trace his way back from the manifest and myriad to an originary unity that gives form to life without deliberate action.

In this he is informed by an ancient Daoist cosmogonic vision, "the three gives birth to the myriads" (*san sheng wanwu* 三生万物).[28] What does this mean? Zhang explains with reference to an "axial age" (800–200 BCE) metaphysics that he believes (with lots of evidence) informs the logic of the medical classics. This was an era when many thinkers proposed versions of how cosmic becoming works. Zhang cites early sources as follows:

> The *Book of Changes* and the *Dao De Jing*, as well as the esoteric alchemical Daoists, spoke of how to let original qi return to non-action: "the Dao gives birth to the One, the One gives birth to Two, the Two gives birth to Three [the yinyang generative dynamic], and the Three gives birth to all the myriad things." Here, One is original qi, Two is yin and yang, and the visceral systems, qi and blood can be understood as the human body's myriad things. If you seek to let the human body's original qi return to a state of non-action, this is a way of letting the myriad things return spontaneously to oneness; only if there is a return to the One can original qi achieve non-action. This process is what the old Daoists called "the latter heaven returning to the former heaven" [or environmental experience returning to the innate source].[29]

Dr. Zhang's cosmogonic understanding of how bodily phenomena arise from original qi (*yuanqi* 元气), along with his unstated understanding that original qi has a deep-seated home and functions as a wellspring, source, or unmoved mover, in the ever-active body,[30] invites a kind of diagnostic leap, a profound sort of clinical thought that reaches far beyond "evidence" to grasp something essential about the life of bodies—each body, each situation. But, when we look at the book from which I have been translating these prefatory remarks, we can see that Zhang himself sees the importance of tracing Dao to its source as more manifest in his classical-cum-contemporary design of formulas and drugs than in the abstractions of ancient philosophy. In his book, he wants to show us how the "vital machine" (*shenji* 神机) found turning through the medical classics is most helpful as a guide to the mundane management of cases, as they transform, manifesting in both changing pathology and a return to health. For him, cases and formulas are a privileged form of thought, one that concretely "traces Dao to its source."[31]

Correlation: Ordering the Manifest and the Myriad

As noted, even ignorant patients, like me, have their hunches and stories about what's really going on inside their bodies, in the invisible dark, back toward the "original sources" of suffering. But the kind of medical knowing that sees a certain order in all those images, and links the manifestations to their hidden roots in more unitary "original" processes, is disciplined. The doctor's perception becomes medically conceptual (Chairman Mao might say) when he links the results of the four examinations to the analytical systems—in writing about figure 1 I refer to them as methods of discernment—available in the Chinese medical archive.[32] I will show that these analytics are preeminently *correlative* and *classificatory*. As such, they rely on conventional (or traditional) kinships and distinctions, mobilizing several great systems of natural linkage and discontinuity.

We can approach this so-called correlative science by listing a few of the "pattern-discerning" disciplines that are popular in clinics of Chinese medicine these days, and then showing them at work in a description of a well-known pattern of disorder. Here are some of the analytic systems that are ready-to-hand for the Chinese doctor: eight rubrics, four sectors, six channels, visceral systems, and *jing/ qi/blood*.[33] One of these we already have some hunches about, after having seen the five visceral systems outlined in table 1 (chapter 2). That table summarizes the network connections traditionally associated with each of the five great visceral systems and gives you an idea of the kind of correlations and distinctions that might be invoked as clinical understanding moves from the perceptible image to the underlying systematic process. It would be rare, however, to analyze a presenting illness with reference only to visceral systems. Consider, for example, some of the conventional correlations of six of the eight rubrics, an analytic technique that is almost always used (box 4).

Just about any sign can be classified as cool or warm, shallow or deep, repletion or depletion, yin or yang. And though the classifications of facts collected in the four examinations, sorted as falling under one or another of the eight rubrics, is sometimes intuitively obvious—a fever and dry mouth are clearly warm and yang— basically the correlations are conventional and traditional. In Maoist idiom, they arise from the "several thousand years of recorded experience of the masses' struggle against disease." And they need to be memorized by the medical student and kept in mind by the practitioner. These known lists of correlations are a resource for the doctor's thinking.

Let's get just a little closer to actual clinical work with an example: suppose the patient presents with some "heart" symptoms, such as palpitations. A correlation to the heart visceral system is easy to guess, but this initial hunch doesn't take you very far. Because the visceral systems are not confined to the heart organ itself, the observation of a heart system pathology only enhances your curiosity about other expressions of a possibly more deep-seated disorder. Taking the pulse, you note that the qualities of pulsation are "slender" and "weak" (these conventionally, by correlation, tell you to

Box 4. Eight Rubrics Correlations

Cool and Warm Symptoms

Cool: clenching; withdrawn and taciturn; stiffness; pale face and lips; tongue coating white, thin; tongue pale; sleepy; clear urine; likes warm food; pulse sunken, small, moderate . . .

Warm: stretching/reaching; fluid movements; agitation and restlessness; reddish face, lips, nails; staring eyes; dry mouth and lips; rough dry yellow tongue coating; thick yellow mucus; thirsty; constipation; pulse floating, swollen, accelerated, forceful . . .

Shallow and Deep Symptoms

Shallow: intolerance of cold, slight fever, head and body aches, stuffy nose, pain in limbs; tongue coating white; pulse floating . . .

Deep: high fever, agitation, thirst, chest or abdominal pain, constipation or diarrhea, scant reddish urination; tongue coating yellow or gray; pulse sinking . . .

Depletion and Repletion Symptoms

Qi Depletion: shortness of breath, cold extremities, dizziness, ringing in ears, etc.

Qi Repletion: stuffy chest, upset stomach, nausea, hectic fever and delirium, etc.

Blood Depletion: paleness, agitation, night fevers, cramps, depleted fluids, etc.

Blood Repletion: localized swelling and pain, acute abdominal pain, distensions, black stools, etc.

(Similar depletion/repletion correlations can be listed for each of the five visceral systems.)

Yin and Yang Symptoms

(These correlations follow the first three sets according to the initiating and completing logic of yang and yin, but the lists of symptoms would be much longer. This fourth couple of the eight rubrics is thus omitted here for simplicity.)

---

expect that qi and blood are both depleted), and you might also note the confirming fact that the patient's face is pale, nearly gray. Looking at the tongue, you observe that the body of the tongue is unusually pale, a sign you can correlate under the rubrics "depletion" and "cold" (recall that these are two of the eight rubrics, box 4). If the tongue coating is at the same time white, this indicates again that qi and blood might be simultaneously depleted. Invoking qi and blood, we can see that the *jing*/qi/blood method of discerning a pattern is also brought to bear. Eight rubrics classifications have shown that this is not such a deep-seated disorder that *jing*-essence would be considered to be affected, and the signs that would correlate with blood depletion are not present. At about this point you will be thinking that since "the heart rules the blood and the vessels" and "vents at the tongue" and "manifests in the face" (table 1), you have pretty much landed on a rather straightforward pattern: "heart qi depletion."[34] Here's a standard description of this pattern:

> Pattern of heart qi depletion: Heart throbbing or palpitations, easily startled, difficulty sleeping, forgetfulness, facial color pale and white, little energy and halting speech, spontaneous sweating, vital exhaustion and lack of vigor, white tongue coating, pale tongue color, pulse slender and weak.[35]

Then when you turn to the asking examination, you can perhaps impress the patient by asking whether he is often forgetful, perspires for no reason, or has difficulty sleeping. Hearing these questions, patients sometimes ask, "How did you know?"

Well, how did you know? Perhaps from having memorized masses of correlations and being fast on your feet as you classify, together and apart, the miscellaneous signs presented by the patient. With your correlational work, you determine that the syndrome is *not* (yet) deep-seated in (for example) the blood storage functions of the liver system, and that a general pattern of exhaustion is more due to a shortfall of yang stimulus than to a buildup of sluggish yin substance. The pattern identified is now well characterized by correlation, but it also has been discerned as a dynamic situation: cooling affects excessive warmth, relatively shallow symptoms can go deep, repletion in one system can lead to depletion in another, and, of course, yang stimulus seeks completion in yin stabilities. These processual tendencies are well understood by clinicians (though here I am only noting an eight rubrics version of pathological process, far simpler than the sophisticated understanding of most TCM clinicians). The correlations made by the many methods of discerning patterns set up a dynamic situation, a pattern of emerging and changing disorders, that invites a parallel therapeutic intervention, ready to change course in its path downward and inward as it traces qi to its source.

Patterns of disorder are very numerous indeed, almost infinite in theory. Even the conventionally used methods of discerning patterns are too many, in a sense. Every pattern-discerning practitioner must navigate among many effective and overlapping options to arrive at a set of correlations and names—a pattern—that persuades him and the patient. Like "heart qi depletion" or "spring warm repletion in the yang visceral systems" (see box 2), patterns are discerned and named in a way that shows them — to those who know — to be convergences and expressions of more general processes. And these processes, known as physiology and pathology in modern Chinese medicine, must be understood if there is to be any successful interruption of a disordered flow, any effective way of nudging the body toward better health.[36]

Conclusion

I began this chapter with a proverb drawn from a very early source, the fifth-century *Book of the Later Han*: "Medicine is thought" (*yizhe yi ye* 医者意也). Though there is reason to believe that this formula has been invoked from time to time in the long history of Chinese medical argumentation, it recently was made salient again by a writer of Chinese medical history and theory, Liao Yuqun. *Medicine Is Thought* is the title of his 2006 book subtitled *Knowing Chinese Medicine*. Here is part of this modern author's comment on the classical texts:

Following Guo Yu's time [first century CE, when he argued that failures to cure happen mainly when thinking is absent], a famous master of the Southern Dynasty, Tao Hongjing (456–536 CE) articulated rather early that medicine is thought. "Thus it was that Tao intimated, medicine is thought. Those who were known as good doctors of old, because they applied limits to their capacity for thinking, they were able to know and treat the sick. All their thoughts arose from the moment, so they didn't woodenly adopt traditional formulas to treat the illness."[37]

By implication, then, the great doctors of the past crafted every medical formula and strategy in the moment to fit the particular pattern they were able to discern through responsive and imaginative thought. The modern author of this philological discussion notes that, for the ancients, "thinking" (*yi* 意) meant, above all, perceptiveness. Yet "they applied limits to their capacity for thinking"; they disciplined their imaginations. Chinese medicine's tools of perception and conception are very rich but not infinitely so, and they are limited on purpose, this classic source seems to say. The author goes on:

> Summarizing the above, it was really after the Song Dynasty that doctors frequently pointed out that "medicine is thought." The *Imperial Grace Formulary of the Taiping Shengguo Period* 太平圣惠方, 992 CE) lays it out as follows: "Yes, medicine is thought! Illness is born on the inside and medicines adjust the condition (*tiao* 调) from the outside. Doctors illuminate the pattern (*mingli* 明理) of illness, and medicines act on it like a god (*rushen* 如神). This magical efficacy arises from engagement with the sorts of phenomena, and from minute participation in the transformations and the Changes (*bianyi* 变易)." This is the Way of subtlety, the very limit of thought in use.[38]

This brilliant summation from more than a thousand years ago completes the point around which this chapter has been circling. Moreover, because it cannot do otherwise for a pragmatist, it also leads us toward chapter 4 on the nature of human medical action. The authorities quoted in this chapter want to assure us that, yes, the work of medicine is inseparable from the practice of thinking. Just as it is written in the *Sacred Remedies*, pathology has its genesis on the inside of our bodies, but it expresses itself in signs on the surface, and these signs gather in manifest and reported human experience. Medicines, on the other hand, are brought to bear from the outside to adjust the course of the illness process. It is the doctor's job to perceptively grasp the pattern of disorder, and if he does, the herbal medicines he or she composes can magically alter the pathological process. The healer's effectiveness arises from an intimate grasp of the traditional correlations and classifications, and from deep attentiveness to the unceasing transformations of living experience. This Way brings us near to the subtlest things, and it is fundamentally pragmatic. Medicine is the limit case of thought in use.

4

Action: Practice, Roots, Ethics

摸着石头过河

Let's cross the river by feeling for stones.

Deng Xiaoping, early Reform Period

In medicine, action, or, perhaps I should say, actionability, is the criterion of value, both for things and thoughts. This is true of any modern medicine. Antisepsis and antibiotics, as they became foundations of public health action in the twentieth century, were tools that made bacteria into the most real of real things, and bacteriological thought placed hygiene, microscopy, immunization, and infectious disease control at the center of the way "Western medicine" legitimized itself and declared its truth. The Pasteurian microbe's long and complex path to an unchallenged existence as an agent of disease was possible mainly because its proponents were able to show how human aims could be better served when this kind of object was discerned and brought under control.

There are many factors that can be said to cause disease, and the explanatory story differs from case to case. Causation is always "multifactorial." But for classic magic bullet biomedicine, proliferations of certain bacteria in human bodies have a special value because they became, quite recently, the most efficient point at which to intervene in a causal chain or actor network.[1] The microbe, a gathered thing, is known to be "the cause" of the affliction. As historians of science have demonstrated again and again, the human bio-agent is a thing constructed in the context of practice (but it is no less real for all that).[2] Practice in medical research is partly guided by the relatively arbitrary conventions of existing knowledge. Paradigms and thought styles can be conservative about the factual and the salient.[3] And medical things and thoughts—unlike fictional characters and contemplative philosophies—must actively and ethically serve the ends desired by particular human beings.

As its practitioners sought to legitimate traditional Chinese medicine (TCM) in a world committed to scientific development, it is little wonder that they turned first to arguments about efficacy. Under attack from modernizing scientizers since the 1920s, practitioners of Chinese medicine still fight for their right to practice medicine by calling on a powerful common tool, the argument—or perhaps it's only a reminder to those who already know—that Chinese medicine *works*.[4] Though many moderns around the world don't really think this is true, that vast number of sufferers who have used the methods and herbals of TCM, in the world's most populous nation, are persuaded in their very bodies that TCM does indeed work. It is admitted, of course, that herbs, acupuncture needles, massage, and surface manipulations are not magic bullets, and in practice doctors and patients acknowledge that there are some serious ailments these TCM technologies do not reach well. But patients who have been successfully treated for digestive disorders, pain syndromes, infertility, depression, chronic fatigue, menstrual disorders, anxiety, deafness, and more have unequivocally benefited from the action of TCM's array of agents. These patients tell us that TCM *must be* scientific *because* it works.

But the more sophisticated advocates of Chinese medicine's social and biological value cannot rest with this kind of commonsense assumption. I suggested in chapter 1 that medicine anywhere is more an art than a science, but this too is not a comfortable or logical resting place for advocates of TCM. Many who write about the current state of affairs in TCM want to insist that the field is scientific, and they devote considerable attention to defining the science of TCM in terms of its objectivity (*keguanxing* 客观性), its rationality (*lixing* 理性), or its systematicity (*xitongxing* 系统性). But they also recognize, sometimes helplessly, that real disagreements about the value of an "alternative" medicine center on the reality of the things on which and with which it *acts*. As Zhang Dong notes in the preface to his book *Original Qi, Vital Machine* (appendix 2), no amount of laboratory research using the methods of "modern medicine" can understand the things known to the medicine of early China. Trying to translate the viscera and circulation tracks written about in the *Yellow Emperor's Inner Canon* into the blood vessels and hormones of biomedicine will yield only "imaginary things," objects not worth thinking about. Yet Zhang's book is not only philosophical and methodological critique, it is strongly oriented toward practice, it seeks to guide clinical action now and tomorrow. To that end, he places some of the far-from-imaginary things that make TCM work—original qi, for example—at the center of his argument, and he insists as well that "[practical] medicine is thought."

This chapter will look back at the problem of the real but unfamiliar things discussed in chapter 2 (ontology), and it will reconsider forms of Chinese medical thought, considered in chapter 3, as knowing practice (a pragmatic epistemology). Looked at from the point of view of imperative action—administering the antibiotic, excising the tumor, cooling heart system yang excess—only certain things are salient, and not just anything can be thought. For the medical arts, action is the criterion of value, determining what things we can perceive and what thoughts are to the point. And medical action itself, I will argue eventually, is inseparable from a human-centered ethics.

Stones and Flow

But first let's cross the river by feeling for stones. This is a proverbial formula for everyday practice that is often heard among speakers of modern Chinese. President Deng Xiaoping, as he took the helm of the Chinese state in the late 1970s and began to replace cultural revolution and Maoist-Leninist Thought with an explicit modernizing pragmatism, favored homely proverbs like this chapter's epigraph in selling his reforms to the public. There is a kind of "let's get on with it" tone to such homilies, and quite often in those years (as now) the official imaginary of progress, modernization, development, and economic growth went without saying.[5]

I arrived in Guangzhou to study Chinese medicine just a few years into the Dengist period, and thus it was no accident that my teachers so often emphasized "practice" (*shijian* 实践) to me. When I asked questions about the things, thoughts, and actions I found confusing in textbooks, they would say, "We take practice and experience to be our guides." In one sense, they were encouraging me to get my feet wet with TCM, spend time in clinics figuring out how clinical decisions are actually made and learning to read the things that speak so eloquently to the experts, such as a strung pulse image or a greasy tongue coating. Perhaps they were also just a little skeptical about the truth value of the systematic information I was memorizing in textbooks.

Heeding their sage advice, I began to see my teachers, clinicians all, as experts in making their way across treacherous rivers of illness and finding their footing through "reforming" institutions with precious little guidance from any higher-order narrative.[6] TCM laboratory science had yielded few results at the time, and tradition—that is, the Chinese medical archive—offered far too many choices of strategy. It was not easy to get the job done and serve the people in a way that could be collectively approved.[7] Maoism had made truth into a resultant of class struggle (and thus a political issue). The standard Chinese dictionary definition of "truth" at the time supplied this sentence as its usage example: "absolute truth is nothing more than the sum of all relative truths—Mao Zedong." But whose truth should be included in the "all" of this vision? Who should do the summing? Following what changing rules? And to what ends?

Medicine in 1980s China was required to find its way in the flow of practice at a particularly slippery time. Consider this chapter's epigraph: neither the Chinese nor its English translation quite captures the experience of finding one's way through uncertainty to a desired destination in practice. If this proverb is read too narrowly, one might miss the feeling of bare feet groping along the unstable bottom of a rushing stream, its waters hiding from our sight the contours of the *things*—those partly obscured stones—that demand such nervous care. Knowledge of the situation, a sense of the terrain, is sketchy under circumstances of rapid flow. Imagine the dangers of this operation, as you negotiate your footing on objects that provide no stable ground and in flowing water that nudges you downstream with possibly treacherous currents. At first, when you're standing on the bank looking at the water's surface, most streams would seem to afford many crossing points. But once you've tentatively taken a step or two into the water, your options for ways of fording the stream are progressively reduced. No amount of good thinking or advance planning is going to guarantee safe arrival on the other bank. With your eyes wide open but still half blind, you have to commit yourself to a course of action, one step at a time. As you go you must live with the consequences of each step—the right foot choosing to rely on a downstream stone makes another possible foothold upstream, more to the left, unfeasible forever. Possibly, as you pick your way across the stream, you would reconsider your destination: why, again, did I want to be on that other shore? But this uncertainty can usually be answered confidently. One doesn't often have much choice about the destination, whether it is the bus stop needed for a daily commute, or an effective prescription designed for an uncomfortable illness.

Like any good Chinese proverb, this one can be unfolded even further, and I will return to it in what follows. But I have not yet made the character of Chinese medical action very clear, so let me now turn to a description of the TCM clinical encounter. This mundane event, repeated many times daily throughout East Asia, is not unlike crossing the stream by feeling the stones. We can learn much about practice and action from attending to it.

Action in the Clinic

The clinical encounter of Chinese medicine is most often conducted by fully clothed people with minimal technology and in crowded rooms with little privacy. It often includes a lot of talking and a little touching. Usually doctor and patient face each other, seated at a corner of a desk where the doctor can reach the patient's wrist in order to take her pulse. Family members often hover nearby. In big clinics students and interns are also there, pens and notebooks or computer keyboards at the ready to record symptoms, diagnosis, and drug formulas. This arrangement of bodies expresses the fundamental social composition of the modern clinical encounter, which in

Chinese is referred to as *kanbing*, looking at illness. In these sparsely furnished offices, doctor and patient and their allies look at illness together. Everyone is close to equal in their orientation to the problem, but they are far from identical in their expertise.

When you arrive at a sizable hospital or clinic (one that has a revolving medical staff for TCM services and can authorize health insurance payments, for example), you register at the front desk, asking for the clinic of a particular doctor. Registration fees are high for senior doctors, lower for recent graduates and residents. Though most insurance plans don't pay the full fee, registration is not expensive except for the most famous doctors. (The highest amount I have seen is several thousand RMB, or about three hundred dollars. Registration fees can be as low as five dollars, however.) If you don't already know which doctor you want to see, or if you are not sure who is on duty in clinic today, you can study the picture display of practitioners and their specialties, with their clinic days, hours, and fees, posted inside the front door of the hospital. Then you register at the registration desk for that doctor, that clinic, paying your fee in advance. Part of that fee goes toward paying the doctor's salary.

Registration usually means that you receive a tiny slip of paper or some other record with your unique number for the day on it. Leaving the lobby, you carry it with your personal case record booklet and, sometimes, reports of test results to the clinic you chose. Unceremoniously entering your doctor's busy room—where there are already patients, family members, students, and interns standing around and taking up all the seats—you leave your registration number on his desk, or give it to an assistant. Then you wait, probably in the hallway, probably feeling miserable—you are, after all, a sick person—until your number or name is called from inside the room.

At the point when you are finally able to occupy the patient's chair, facing the doctor across a corner of the table, several key gestures are made. In the consultation rooms of my 1980s field research, and in some clinics still, the doctor or an assistant attaches your registration number on its paper slip to a blank prescription form. More recently, with computers in the clinic, a student or intern or other assistant will open a clinic visit record, entering your registration number and starting to fill out a form that includes space for an herbal prescription.

Think about the meaning of this gesture. Not a word has passed between you and the doctor, he has barely even glanced up from finishing the prescription he's written for the last patient. And yet in starting a prescription form uniquely for you, he promises, and you know, that something will be done. Everyone expects an action to result from this episode of looking at illness together, at least in the form of an herbal medicine prescription. Neither of you is waiting upon lab results to confirm that you are ill. There is no danger that you will be told to go home and just carry on because it's all in your head. In the Chinese medical clinic, there are no purely imaginary illnesses. Both you and your doctor presume that everything is not right with you, *if you say so*. And both of you are confident that there will be some things in the vast Chinese pharmacopeia or arsenal of acupuncture techniques that can address the problem you have presented. Even if you're only feeling just a bit subnormal (and this "subhealth" is a recognized thing, by the way, *ya jiankang* 亚健康), you both know there are powers that can be deployed in the clinic to at least tune you up and make everything work a little better.

The second key gesture that inaugurates the clinical encounter is even more obvious and even more important for determining what will follow. The doctor begins by asking, "Where is your discomfort? What's wrong with you just now?" Your answer might be simple: stomach aches, insomnia, uncontrollable weeping, constipation, shoulder pain. Or it might be more complex and involve telling a story: "I've seen so many different kinds of doctors for these digestive problems, only a few of the things they recommended had any effect but I still have episodes," and so on. The notes recorded in case record booklets and in hospital files, however much they vary in the habits of senior doctors, almost always include some reference to this self-reported "chief complaint." The chief complaint is not a diagnosis of disease nor is it a pattern of disorder, the *zhenghou* discussed in previous chapters. It is, however, the *bing* of *kanbing*, the illness that is looked at in the clinic from all the various points of view in play. This is the thing that sets the aims of action in the TCM clinic, the *bing* illness that presents with the patient and becomes the target of intervention. As she tacitly agrees to the patient's view of pathology, or listens to his assessment of what's wrong now, the doctor expresses the unquestioned ethical stance of traditional medicine: it is the individual desires of the sufferer that identify the problem to be solved.[8]

Having embarked on a TCM consultation, the two of you, doctor and patient, open various lines of communication by means of "the four examinations" (see box 3). Possibly you have carried your case record booklet into the clinic with you, and your doctor, if she is seeing you for the first time, may scan its notes from previous clinical encounters in other places, with other doctors. The doctor or an assistant will find a blank page in your booklet or initiate a computer record, and often someone jots down the signs and symptoms you report as the doctor's queries lead you through the categories of the "four examinations" of "looking, listening/ smelling, asking, and touching." Your pulse and tongue image speak tellingly to the expert

examiner; your stance, coloring, gestural animation, and voice quality give him clues about the state of your energy and nourishment;
and your reports of the ups and downs of your physical experience
over the last days and weeks will begin to suggest a dynamic that can
be analyzed.

Some of this process was presented in chapters 2 and 3 and diagrammed in figure 1. As I argued at length in *Knowing Practice,* the
perceptive collection of signs of illness and the analysis of symptoms
using several different "traditional" systems are best thought of as
forms of action. Some of this action is mental, which is to say (*pace*
Hacking), it is more than representing, it is intervening: forceful,
disciplined, and consequential.[9] The four examinations, for example,
in practice yield far too much information (see box 3). Pulse touching alone can show the complexity of the situation: the possibility
of feeling one or several of twenty-eight pulse images, at several of
eighteen possible points on two slim wrists, is emblematic of the
choices that must be made. Not even trained perception yields a
simple and straightforward picture or a clean category of disease. No
TCM clinician pretends to be alert to all of the possibilities. Most
tend to restrict their touch to a salient few pulse images in a few
especially significant spots (shallow or deep, proximal to or farther
from the thumb, correlated with spleen or kidney systems but not
all five viscera, and so on). This choosing is a form of action that
looks ahead to the discernment of a pattern to come. The pattern
of disorder arrived at through analysis is not the same as the "chief
complaint" reported when our patient sat down with his doctor. Nor
is it an ontological disease. It is, rather, an actionable name for what
is going wrong.

In many TCM clinics, the *kanbing* encounter ends with the
production of an herbal prescription, a *yaofang* (药方). (See box 5

Box 5. The Romance of the Herbal Prescription: *Yaofang* (药方)

Anthropologist Mei Zhan opens her book *Other-Worldly*, an ethnographic study of Chinese medicine in today's world, with her mother's discovery, among her grandfather's effects, of herbal prescriptions written in the 1980s by a well-known senior Chinese doctor, He Yiren. Handwritten on pink hospital stationery, these "*gaofang*" (膏方) included a "diagnostic narrative" of the patient's condition, a long list of plant and animal drugs, and instructions for making them into a medicinal paste for oral consumption. Of course, Mei Zhan was delighted to receive these historical artifacts, which materially connected her and her research to the rich social and natural world gathered together in Chinese medical practice as it pertained to a member of her own family. Her mother was also thrilled that she had found these old documents from several clinical encounters twenty years before. Both mother and daughter saw these documents as condensations of a great deal of history and experience, inseparable from the life and body of father and grandfather, as well as intrinsic to the historical importance of a senior doctor with whom they still had connections. Zhan writes, "The arrival of Dr. He's gao-fang was a moment that saw disparate routes tangled up, unlikely intersections rendered visible, origins relocated and made to multiply, temporalities re-shuffled, and an ethnography that was about to close . . . reopened and plotted anew."[a]

Of course, an appreciation of the many possible meanings of these documents would not result from any straightforward act of reading. It takes considerable skill to design an herbal prescription as the culmination of a *bianzheng lunzhi* process (see figure 1). The prescription in itself contains a great deal of detailed information about the medical condition presented and analyzed. Any well-trained doctor, when an earlier prescription is brought to his attention, can "read back" from that record to see the illness phenomena that were presented in another clinic at some previous time. And up until very recently the act of handwriting a prescription, in sometimes beautiful and sometimes illegible calligraphy, in the presence of the patient and his family, has been understood as the practical and intellectual heart of every clinical encounter.

Mei Zhan is not the only anthropologist to notice the centrality and symbolic force of written *yaofang* (in her case, *gaofang*), but she may be one of the few who has highlighted the romance of the herbal prescription in a published ethnography. Colin Garon, writing from his field research in Beijing clinics, has noted in an unpublished paper that even young trainees in TCM today point out that certain fine points of formula design and medical thinking are lost when the computerized pharmacy imposes its own rules to generate a printed prescription.[b] Even in today's clinics, the work of writing down a thoughtfully designed yaofang is surrounded often by a kind of hush as the doctor concentrates on the array of drug names and quantities unfolding under his hand.

Yaofang are not only a particular expression of one doctor's brilliance and habits of thought; they are not only a sign of strong medicine acting directly; they are also deeply felt reflections or representations of the power, beneficence, and esoteric insight of medicine in general. They too demonstrate what so many like to say: medicine—even the most literal list of medicines—is thought. Anthropologist Jun Wang recognized this complexity in her historical ethnography of modern Chinese medicine. Wang's dissertation argues, with a wide variety of instances, that practices of writing have always been, and still remain, central to the work of TCM. As she conducted interviews and archival research concerning the life of TCM's most prominent modern historian, Ren Yingqiu, she was sometimes presented with

continued

herbal prescriptions he had written: "*fangzi*" (方子) on crumbling slips of hospital paper that had been lovingly saved by his patients, students, and family members. "When the patient took his fangzi to a drugstore, or to see a different Chinese doctor for further treatment, the fangzi was the face of the doctor," she explains.[c] In other words, all the complex authority assembled by famous doctors and their allies (students, teachers, writings, and the medicinals themselves) was gathered and condensed on one small slip of paper, with its handwritten list, not a piece of trash to be lightly discarded.

In her dissertation Wang recounts an occasion in 1998, after her fieldwork was finished, when an old friend facing a complex cancer revealed that she herself had once been treated by Ren Yingqiu.[d] Without much digging in her files, this friend was able to find the original prescription forms, probably written in the early 1980s. The friend and her four visitors all marveled at the neat and masterful calligraphy of these precious historical documents. The *yaofang* seemed to connect all of them, but especially the friend with a recurring cancer, to a respected elder who had died in 1984. At the same time, this group of contemporary companions all wondered whether they could find a doctor as good for the present condition that was threatening their friend's life. And they saw the beauty of the writing itself as the strongest index of Ren Yingqiu's brilliant authority.

a. Zhan, *Other-Worldly*, ix–xi.

b. Garon, "Clinical Concrescences."

c. Wang, *Life History of Ren Yingqiu*, 7. Wang also notes that museums of the history of Chinese medicine invariably display the handwritten prescriptions of famous doctors, many of them fairly recent, but no less respected for being only a few decades old.

d. Ibid., 188.

for a consideration of the rich culture surrounding herbal medicine prescriptions in China.) Nowadays this would most likely be a computer printout listing between four and twenty drugs, proportionally arranged and with quantities specified, all of which can be found in the hospital pharmacy. Sometimes there are brief instructions for preparing the herbal decoction, or "soup," that will be drunk. Carried to the pharmacy, the prescription becomes several piles of drugs that are gathered from many labeled drawers, combined in the proper proportions and wrapped into packets, one for each day you will be taking the medicine.

Especially if you are seeing a TCM doctor for a stubborn chronic complaint (and this is quite usual in today's Chinese clinics), you will be encouraged to prepare and take the medicine at home, monitor your symptoms, and come back in a few days or a week to discuss drug effects, changes in your condition, remaining problems—all the manifestations of the ongoing "birthing and transforming" of effects that is natural to both physiology and pathology.[10] There will always be something, however superficial, to report, and your doctor will always have an idea of how to alter his strategy in a way that continues to nudge your life toward health, toward an end of that chief complaint that you have brought to him and his assistants.

Have a Need? We Will Respond.

In this account of how "looking at illness" (*kanbing*) takes place in Chinese medical clinics, I have emphasized some ordinary gestures and dispositions, and described the down-to-earth conditions that everyone knows they will find in a TCM clinic.[11] Patients do not go to a Chinese doctor expecting an MRI or an angiogram. They may bring lab results, X-ray images, or sonogram snapshots with them, but they expect these kinds of information to be translated into a "more traditional" idiom in the hands of the doctor. As patients, our general expectation is that we can sit down with an experienced expert in "doubtful, difficult, and complex illnesses" (*yinan zabing* 疑难杂病), have our stubborn discomforts attended to, and go away with a collection of medicines that both of us, doctor and patient, feel sure will have some effective results. Not a magic bullet, but a starting point or a step along the way toward a lasting improvement.

People's confidence that action in the clinic will be effective in some way, even though some ailments are rather intractable, has always reminded me of the banner signs one sees in Buddhist and Daoist temples all over China: "Whatever you are seeking, we will respond" (*youqiu bi ying* 有求必应). Gods in Chinese temples have many ways of speaking—through divination techniques, or through monks or nuns willing to interpret the results of divining, or with action that quickly or slowly intervenes in your life, or by bringing good luck with amulets containing prayers. But this banner is perhaps their most direct voice. And it makes a very firm promise.

Chinese medicine makes a similar promise. At the end of chapter 3 I quoted a modern theorist quoting a tenth-century philosophical work, as follows:

> Yes, medicine is thought! Illness is born on the inside and medicines adjust it (*tiao* 调) from the outside. Doctors illuminate the pattern (*mingli* 明理) of illness, and medicines act on it like a god (*rushen* 如神). This magical efficacy arises from engagement with the sorts of phenomena, and from minute participation in the transformations and the Changes (*bianyi* 变易). This is the Way of subtlety, the very limit of thought in use.[12]

This paragraph is an effective and polemical summary of the sophisticated self-image that has emerged in recent decades among thoughtful Chinese medicine practitioners. At the very least, this citation of a traditional text, by Liao Yuqun, makes it impossible to separate thought, or mental representation, from action, or compassionate intervention. The message is the same as that of the gods in our local temple, to whom we bring our chief complaints. "Can you make your need clear?" they ask; can it be "illuminated"? If you're asking for help, "we must respond," at least with an "adjustment" of your fate.

Medical action, which "adjusts from outside" the pathology illuminated as a pattern of disorder (see the examination and discernment process, figure 1), is here compared to the magical efficacy, the *ling* (灵) powers, of the gods.[13] A shared or distributed agency is claimed for medical action. Doctors illuminate the pattern (and this "illumination" is made up of the words for luminous vision, *ming*, and patterned reasoning, *li*), but doctors are not the only agents at work. Medicines—natural drugs with their long history of known powers—act too, in collaboration with medical thought.

Liao Yuqun admits little doubt about the ability of medicines to "adjust" illness.[14] If you have a need—a pathology with particular characteristics, a *zhenghou*, a pattern of disorder—we godlike medicines will respond, specifically, to what ails you, with our warming or tonifying, our heart-calming or stomach-sweetening capacities. This confidence about medicine's ability to alter a bad situation is quite widespread. Carla Nappi's study of Li Shizhen, the seventeenth-century chronicler of China's materia medica, has rediscovered the capacity of the medicinals known to the herbal tradition to participate in constant change, to express their own nature in transformative ways.[15] In recent research among herbalists in China's southwestern provinces, moreover, Lili Lai and I have talked with many healers who gather medicine in the mountains. They express deep respect for the plants and other natural things they study and use, believing that for every human complaint there is, somewhere in China's wilder places, a natural agent that can influence pathological process, "adjust" its course in a human body and a life. And the senior Chinese doctors staffing public and private hospitals and clinics in China's cities also know that it is part of their job to express easy confidence in their methods. This is part of clinical communication. A knowing practitioner's smiling reassurances recruit the patient's compliance and increase her willingness to work through a healing process, even if it involves swallowing a lot of nasty-tasting soups. (See appendix 1, "Comparison and Causation," for related points.)

But of course, "the transformations and the changes" are myriad, reality comes to us as a dizzying array of things, all of which are active and transforming—like Zhuangzi's bugs and leopards, like Lu Guangxin's thing-images we face (*duixiang* 对象, see chapter 2). The myriad things, constantly birthing and transforming, throwing up ten thousand images from invisible sources, are rather like water flowing over unseen rocks. Perhaps these things—knee pain and tongue images, case histories and constipation—are both the water *and* the rocks, the uneven reality across which we must feel our way, doctors and gods seeking that other shore of better health and a less disastrous fate.

This confusing flow of practice is why, Liao Yuqun assures us here, it is a special kind of expertise to "engage with the sorts."[16] Look again at box 4, which lists the signs and symptoms sorted by the analytic method known as the eight rubrics. With this relatively simple method, medical practitioners learn how to sort signs and symptoms into "rubrics" with the understanding that the resulting groupings of phenomena, the "sorts," will accurately reflect a coherent underlying process. Symptoms tending toward warmth, depletion, interiority, and a yang type of activity, once they are sorted into the conventional rubrics, can be matched to the countering powers of medicines: cooling, nourishing, drawing out, and yin-classified medicines can be gathered and matched to counter and adjust the flow of pathology.[17] Note, then, that there are even more agents in this situation than I have been acknowledging: not only the doctor and his patterning thought; not only the drugs and their storied efficacies; but also the changes and surprises of pathology itself, the patterns that make for a—temporary, we hope—bad fate.

Medicine must respond. The quotation above from Liao Yuqun's book, *Medicine Is Thought,* begins by taking the same form as the promises of the gods. *Have you brought a need* to us, are you presenting in the clinic with a chief complaint? *We will respond,* we have already attached your registration number to a pharmacy form. Moreover, we have special powers, as experienced doctors, first to "illuminate" the pattern of your affliction as it emerges, and then to mobilize the suitable medicines that can act on it "like a god." Like the ranks of gods in the heavenly empire, TCM doctors are not omnipotent or ubiquitous, but they know the transformative powers of their medicines.

But as I argued in chapter 3 with the help of Zhang Dong (appendix 2) and Zhuangzi, this intervention is not entirely "from outside" the body, though Liao suggests as much at first. His ancient author hastens to point out that action "like a god" is made possible by "engagement with the sorts" and "minute participation in the transformations." To maintain the metaphor of this chapter's epigraph, then, it would seem that doctor and patient, clinics and medicines, physiological and pathological processes, are fording that stream together, negotiating and "engaging" the confusions of practice with many things at risk of dissolving, washing away, turning out to be other than expected. So now we should turn to look for more specific efficacies hidden in "the Way of subtlety," the action-form of "thought-in-use."

Five Phases Relativities

It is usual for modern textbooks of TCM to assert that the "theoretical foundations" of the field boil down to two classical systems of thought: the dynamics of yin and yang and the correlative relations of the five phases.[18] In the discussion thus far I have introduced the eight rubrics as one example of how a yinyang logic operates in a process of pattern discernment. At the same time I have emphasized the limits of this kind of disciplined thought: both the way in which various TCM analytics limit what is perceived in the clinical encounter, and the ways in which the living mess of illness spills over all limits imposed by conventional ways of sorting things out. It could be argued that yinyang is both a powerful way of seeing how things happen and too capacious to offer any obvious point of intervention (and thus it could be beside the point for medical action). It takes the arbitrary correlations of a system like the eight rubrics to begin to sort yang from yin, so that counter-matching yin or yang agents can be brought to bear "from outside" against pathological process. But this tidying-up procedure is only the beginning of TCM "thought-in-use."

Consider the five phases: this system of correlations and interactions is also powerful and too capacious. Joseph Needham liked to call the five phases "elements," by analogy to, for example, Galenic medicine, because these correlative groupings are named after commonsense things: wood, fire, earth, metal, and water. But the classic medical writings make it clear that the system is not referring only to solid masses of different types, or even to arbitrarily named "rubrics." The things classified as wood or earth, fire, metal, or water exist and act in relation to each other powerfully. Each of the "phases" has a generative or constraining, injuring or supporting relation with one of the other "phases," so we can see that there are a great many relationships in play in pathophysiological body time.

At first glance a five phases analysis might seem only to add to the confusions of practice. Here's a passage from the "Plain Questions" that demonstrates the difficulty:

> The eastern quarter generates wind, wind generates wood, wood generates sour, sour generates liver, liver generates muscle, muscle generates heart, liver rules the eyes. This process in Heaven is dark generative potential (*xuan* 玄), in humanity is the Dao, on earth is transformation. Transformation generates the five flavors, the Dao generates wisdom, dark potential generates vitality (*shen* 神). Vitality in heaven is wind, on earth is wood, in the human frame is muscle, among the viscera is the liver, among the colors is blue-green, among the musical notes is *jue*, among the inflected tones is *hu*, in movement is grasping, among the orifices is the eyes, among the flavors is sour, and among the intentions is anger. Anger injures liver and sorrow overcomes anger, wind injures muscle and dry overcomes wind, sour injures muscle and pungent overcomes sour.[19]

The passage is clearly archaic, and closely analyzed it would yield many relations that contradict contemporary received wisdom about how the five phases sort the myriad things. Especially for a modern medicine that treats the body largely apart from its environment—modern doctors don't concern themselves overmuch with "the eastern quarter" or the sounds of *jue* and *hu*—this complexity linking wind pathologies and the wood phase, the liver visceral system and sour-flavored things, suggests too many ways in which the things of the world can be brought to bear on my particular illness. But modern five phases systematics imposes a certain order on all these teeming generations and injuries.

Table 1, you will recall, listed some five phases correlations associated with the body's interpenetrating visceral systems. Translating the five yin visceral systems into a five phases logic, we know that the heart system is affiliated with the fire phase, the lung system with metal, the spleen system with earth, the liver system with wood, and the kidney system with the water phase. These affiliations, along with those of other things, such as flavors, colors, sounds, weathers, orifices, and places, are listed in table 2. In theory, in modern five phases use, all the myriad inter-transforming things could be sorted as wood, fire, earth, metal, or water alongside the five yin visceral systems. Of course, this includes those magical medicines, each with its "taste" classification, which act on illness "like a god."

The five groupings achieved by these correlations are only half the story, however. If this were just a typology or classification, it would be static and useless to an activist medicine. For correlations to be medically useful, we must also consider the dynamic relations between the things sorted. As the "Plain Questions" passage above indicates, things of one phase "generate," produce, or give rise to things belonging to a phase "downstream" from it. The modern synthesis holds that "wood" generates "fire," which generates "earth," which generates "metal," which generates "water." And the water phase in turn generates wood phase things.

Table 2. The Correlates of the Five Phases

Five musical tones		Nature						Five phases	Human body							
	Five tastes	Five colors	Five changes	Five weathers	Five regions	Five seasons			Five yin organs	Six yang organs*	Five senses	Body parts	Emotions	Five voices	Actions
Jue	sour	blue	birth	windy	east	spring	wood		liver	gall bladder	eye	sinews	anger	shouting	grasping
Zhi	bitter	red	growth	hot	south	summer	fire		heart	small intestine	tongue	arteries	joy	laughing	nervous
Gong	sweet	yellow	change	humid	center	late summer	earth		spleen	stomach	mouth	flesh	reflection	singing	vomiting
Shang	pungent	white	gathering	dry	west	autumn	metal		lung	large intestine	nose	skin and hair	sadness	crying	coughing
Yu	salty	black	storage	cold	north	winter	water		kidney	urinary bladder	ear	bone	fear	moaning	trembling

Source: Yin, ed., *Basic Theory of Chinese Medicine*, 20.
*The sixth yang organ is the Triple Burner, which involves upper, middle, and lower viscera, so it is not readily correlated with any one yin organ.

The relations of production and restraint are diagrammed in figure 3. If we use this schematic in thinking of clinical cases, we can conclude after some careful analysis that a drug classified as sour, which thus belongs to the wood phase, would have a positive generative effect on heart system deficiencies, because that system is just one phase downstream from "wood" in the production sequence. Similarly, a sour drug might restrain excessive "sweetness" in the earth phase, to which the spleen system belongs.

Working out the action implications of box 4 with the help of figure 3, we would find considerable difficulty in deciding what system, what phase, is the true and proper source of the manifest illness facing us. Which phase should be the target of an intervention? Seen purely logically, influences travel over the arrows in figure 3 far too freely. A heart qi depletion (mentioned in chapter 3) might need to be treated with "productive" wood phase medicines, or it might need to be treated by reducing the excessive "restraint" activity of kidney system water over the heart system. How would the force of water influences be reduced, though? Perhaps by building spleen system earth phase productivity, which would act to restrain kidney water. But as long as heart fire is weakened, I might suspect that spleen earth may be ailing as well because its productive phase "upstream" is depleted. And on and on it goes. Five phases diagnostic logic works in a number of tight circles that present no single cause or source, invite no simple intervention.

Seeking Roots

In considering here the relativities of just one theoretical system, the five phases, I have suggested that a practitioner could easily become overwhelmed with the possibilities of explanation, and

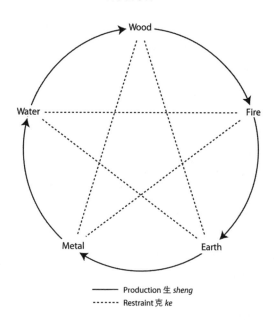

Figure 3. Production and restraint relations of the five phases

thus with the difficult choices that must be made in designing an intervention. Also aware of a huge archive of case records, herbal prescriptions, debates, experiences, experiments, doubts and worries, appealing mythologies, and acts of faith, even experienced doctors might have difficulty developing any clinical certitude.[20] The problems that present to the doctor are very numerous, the analytical resources he can draw on are very rich: even in a very self-conscious twentieth-century literature of medical education, there are no standard rulebooks for responsible action.

Fortunately, doctors, writers, and educators in the world of Chinese medicine have some rules of thumb—one might even call them traditions—that respond to the infiniteness of the transformations and the changes. They tell their students and interns, and they often told me, "To manage illness one must seek out the root" (*zhi-bing bi qiu yu ben* 治病必求于本). Can this search for a "root"—or source, or origin—of pathological process be a way of making action from thought?

There is so much potential for getting it wrong. It is no accident that a significant literature in Chinese medicine, much of it dating from periods before the arrival of Western biomedicine in East Asia, reflects critically on the meaning of therapeutic mistakes. The commentaries published with the many case histories that make up an important category of the historical archive also often highlight the errors of those doctors who attempted a treatment that fell short before the case found its way to our (presumably less muddle-headed) teacher-writer's pharmacy.[21] Quite often the author of a case commentary, justifying his own clinical strategy with a report of the positive outcome in a complex illness, will explain how he found the true root of the ailment presented, after some previous practitioners had adopted the most obvious but only superficial approach.[22]

In Chinese medical education, I don't think anyone ever really explains to the budding clinician how to pull off an identification of *the* root, as the practitioner correlates and infers his way into the darkness of pathological process, or, to mix metaphors, feels his way along the slippery riverbed of chronic illness trying to distinguish between pathological sources and symptomatic expressions. Even when you have a hypothesis about the dynamic sources of the many symptoms you've perceived, how do you know you've found *the* root? How do you know that you are not just imagining your way to some plausible but ultimately bogus process that will not be, in the end, successfully actionable? This uncertainty is one reason medical education is an extended process in China, involving a lot of work as a junior in the clinics of senior doctors, writing case notes at that crowded table. Indeed, those junior clinicians still, in the course of their advanced medical education, are expected to take the day's cases home and make their own copies of symptom lists and prescription formulas. Their clinical teachers encourage them to analyze and reanalyze the logic of each intervention, to relive the unwritten thought process by which an experienced doctor found the root source of a complex pattern and then designed a formula structured to distinguish between the most central aspects and those that are more peripheral.

Deng Tietao, a Guangzhou authority and storied teacher of TCM, attempts a preliminary introduction to the problem of tracing the root in a theoretical foundations text, but even he doesn't explain how to pull off the magic trick of knowing for sure what the root is. He treats it as a technical problem, however, in the hope that experience will guide the student and reader. Here's one of his examples, perhaps especially interesting for those of us who are prone to headaches. He begins his explanation with this:

> "In curing illness seek the root" is a basic principle of the *bianzheng lunzhi* (discerning patterns and determining therapies, see figure 1) system, according to which you must seek out the basic reasons for disease, and advance therapy on the basis of your identification of the illness essence.
>
> Headache, for example, can result from various causes such as an infection, blood depletion, phlegmy dampness, blood stasis, or liver system yang qi flaming upward.[23] In treating it, you need to target its cause, and advance your treatment by distinguishing among [the following parallel treatment methods]: resolving the surface [where the infection is], bolstering blood, drying damp and transforming

phlegm, enlivening blood and transforming stasis, or calming the liver and subduing yang qi.[24]

We can see from this example, with its list of patterns and parallel list of treatment strategies, that the "root" being traced is not a structural foundation of the disease: it is not a lesion, it is not a population of microbes that can be wiped out, it is not a localized trauma in your body. Rather, the root "causes" listed here are all disease processes that have their vicissitudes and involve much of the person's body. (Not just the head, and not just now, when the patient is in your clinic.) A root is a functional source of disorder that changes through time and must be caught in the act of causing human misery.

The clinical imperative of tracing down to the main root, then, is inseparable from time considerations in both pathology and therapeutics. The question of timing is evident in some rules of thumb that Deng derives, following the headache example above. The most important derived principle he explains is called "root and branch, urgent and slow."

> "Root and branch, urgent and slow" refers to the flexible (*linghuo*) deployment of the principle of treating illness by seeking the root.
>   1) if it's urgent, treat the branch symptoms,
>   2) if it's slow, treat the root,
>   3) when needed treat root and branch together.

Just looking at the first of these three directives, we can see that knowing the difference between root and branch phenomena is crucially important. Deng supplies an example to help us see the urgency of keeping these things properly sorted.

(1) when it is urgent, treat the branch—especially if the branch phenomena are life-threatening or making it impossible to treat the root. For example, in a patient with liver disease, who is manifesting severe symptoms of abdominal edema and distension, shortness of breath, and no urination with constipation, you should first resolve the branch phenomenon of abdominal fluids, cause urine and feces to pass out, reduce abdominal distension, and when the condition has stabilized then you can treat the root, which is the liver system.[25]

These medical images of roots and branches arise from seasoned experience in the clinic, even though Deng's written lessons still don't tell medical students how to be sure they have grasped the essential nature of the liver disease from which their patient is probably suffering. But students gradually learn to see things from the perspective of their teachers, experienced clinicians like Deng Tietao. That is, they are taught that they will have to make a distinction, in each case of illness they face, between essence and epiphenomenon, between primary and secondary problems, between roots and branches. Tracing the root requires thought, and as I have noted above, it demands that the infinity of significant manifestations be limited, or be subjected to a sorting process in which we let tradition show us some reliable patterns. Moreover, the things recognized by medicine must also become *salient*, the actionable "images we face" (Lu Guangxin's *duixiang*) under particular conditions. The transformations and the changes can throw up a lot of strange images, but the images actually facing us—these *duixiang* that are present at hand[26]—and the patterns (*li* 理) we recognize in physiology and pathology are that subset of the possible that a practical person might call the actual.

But let's look again at Deng Tietao's rules of thumb about roots and branches. In defining his principles, Deng uses the term *linghuo*, which in medical usage means flexible and agile, responsive and efficacious. This is a word that is often used to describe the talents of the most inspired and respected doctors in traditional medicine. It is a beautiful word, combining *huo*, a word for living, with *ling*, which perhaps most basically means effective. Gods and spirits are *ling* (after all, if you present a need, they must respond); the magical acts they pull off are evidence of their *ling* effectiveness. Medicines are *ling*, too: we have already seen that medicines, properly deployed, can "act like a god." Perhaps this little adjective *linghuo* can be drawn out to remind us that a good doctor is magically lively, an embodiment of effective vitality. Buried in Deng Tietao's rather dry and technical explication of some essential clinical rules of thumb, then, we find a nearly religious attitude toward clinical practice: it can be done not only properly, but brilliantly, magically, if you know how to trace symptomatic experience down to its roots.

Humanity as Root

Now that *linghuo* magical vitality has brought us back to questions of practice, I want to start fulfilling some promises I have been making in this book's wandering argument, promises that I have not yet kept. Most obviously, I have not even broached the topic of ethics announced in the title of this chapter. But I also haven't quite finished with that other modern pragmatist, Deng Xiaoping, who invited us to cross the river by feeling for stones.

Crossing the river by feeling for stones: this pragmatic method of making progress might be the only possible one under present world circumstances. Some philosophical pragmatists might argue that relatively blind groping amidst constant change is in fact the only way any progress is ever made. But this metaphor reexamined also allows us to ask: Why would anyone want to cross the river in the first place? Why is our practitioner aiming to cross *this* stream, to get to *that* other side? Perhaps we should just turn around and go home and forget all metaphors that urge us to risky crossings leading toward barely visible and possibly undesirable other shores.

All kinds of modern Chinese thinkers have asked questions analogous to this. So let me abandon an increasingly flawed metaphor and worry about its more direct implications: there is a stubborn problem with all pragmatic philosophies. They seem to offer no resources for an absolutely correct ethics or an unimpeachable politics. Fully aware that truth is collectively constructed, drowning in the transformations and changes of a vast natural Way, we are thrown back on agnosticism about the nature of any one shared world or universal ethical rulebook: How can we direct our collective human path? Lenin's question looms: What is to be done?[27]

With this question we have finally gotten back to some Terry Lecture religion-and-science dilemmas. I want to conclude, then, by turning again to Lu Guangxin, a Chinese medical authority I have cited several times already. It was Dr. Lu who chose to refer to medical things as *duixiang*, "the image we face." In the 1995 preface to his collected essays, Dr. Lu argues that medicine is fundamentally humanistic. To make this argument, he refers to philosophical and clinical forebears as he makes his way through the pragmatic and relativistic waters of a medical heritage that—as I have tried to show—is far too rich to guide action in any obvious and consensually agreed way. Especially crucial for Dr. Lu's humanism is a line from the famous early twentieth-century philologist and revolutionary Zhang Taiyan, who was also a physician, though he is more remembered for his politics.[28] In his book on modernizing Chinese medicine, Zhang Taiyan said, in 1929, "The Way is not far from humanity, the body of the ill person is its greatest teacher."[29]

Perhaps thinking of that everyday feature of Chinese medical work discussed above, the fact that the chief complaint and reported symptoms of the patient supply the central telos of TCM knowing practice, Lu Guangxin's preface takes up this fascinating observation by Zhang Taiyan and runs with it. In his conclusion to a section called "If the Root Is Sound, the Way Can Come to Life," he touches on many of the things and thoughts I have been trying to make salient:

> The self-health and self-curing capacity of human life-generating qi is the thing we serve and the thing we study.[30] It is the thing through which Chinese medicine researchers must diligently become "great doctors of the masses." Qi is that stuff through which we may become touchstones of genuine Chinese medicine. If we depart from this human life-generating qi, this "root" of life-generation, which must be sought in the nurturing of life and in the treatment of illness, then we medical people cannot expect any genuine Chinese medicine to survive.
>
> Hence the Way of Chinese medicine [advises] "the Way is not far from humanity, let the body (身体 shenti) of the patient be your respected teacher." The root of Chinese medicine's Way, or Dao, is the study of the human: learn from and with the things you serve [e.g., patients, students, bodies]; learn from and with the things on which medicine relies [e.g., drugs, symptoms]; learn from and with the things that develop medicine [e.g., scientific results, historical research];

learn from and with life-nurturance and disease treatment in practice, and seek development *only* out of practice. Medicine at root is humanism.[31]

It would seem that Lu concludes here with a non sequitur. Why is all this engagement with things in practice, like bodies and drugs and books, so obviously humanistic? How can that most general force and form in the cosmos, life-generating qi, bring us so definitively to some root in the (merely) human? We should bear in mind, perhaps, that Lu Guangxin, and the other contemporary authorities I have cited here, writes as a doctor and an activist for traditional Chinese medicine. He also writes as a Maoist populist. In Lu's case in particular, his philosophy tends to adopt an unapologetic political tone: here, for example, he speaks of how we might become "great doctors of the masses." His idiom is thoroughly Maoist, and thus it is typical of him as of others in his generation to insist that we can "seek development only out of practice."[32]

But Zhang Taiyan's advice, cited by Lu, is perhaps even more revealing: "Let the body of the patient be your respected teacher." The modern medical situation constantly speaks its imperative to action. We must grope our way to that other shore of better health because this is what the people need and want, and we must do it with their help. "If the root is sound," Lu Guangxin says, "the Way can come to life." Action begins and ends with a commitment to some part of the ever-changing cosmos, in this case, humanity. A Chinese medical ethics "takes the human to be the root," but because humanity is not far from the Way, a medicine that has all the resources of the universe near at hand—the natural drugs, the case histories, the channels of qi, the patterns of the Changes—can use a vast arsenal to tinker and tweak with pathology, to nudge human lives toward better health. Some experts think of this kind of action as lordly non-action, the famous *wuwei* (无为) of the ancient Daoists (Zhang Dong does, see appendix 2). But whatever the form taken by medical action (traditional or modern, Western or Chinese, Maoist or Daoist), it is through the lens of medical purposes and commitments that thought and things emerge as salient, actual, and true.

Conclusion

I want to conclude with one last polemical remark that gathers a number of the threads I and our various Chinese medical authorities have been weaving together in these lectures. Again, this is Lu Guangxin:

> The proverb "Medicine is thought, reflection on and by human beings" is a practical concept that applies thought to the character of things. Chinese medicine is an opening: "investigate the border between Heaven and the human, penetrate the difference between illness and health, accord with the Way of life giving birth to life—then Heaven and the human cannot but join their powers for the better." This is the effective practical wisdom of a wholesome cosmos in which life ceaselessly gives birth to more life. This is the Way of medicine.[33]

And it is here, on this simultaneously natural and ethical terrain, that we can see how an East Asian science joins its unique powers for knowing and intervening in the patterns of human life and human suffering with the virtues of the myriad things that make up the vast flow of the spontaneous cosmic Way.

For me, for a long time now, Chinese medicine has been an opening to a new and different world of things, thoughts, and actions: it has allowed me to hear deep things talked about, it has made me struggle to understand, it has required close attention to translation, it has been an invitation to understand knowledge as a practice and healing as a mode of existence. I hope these lectures have been a way of sharing with you that problematic thrill, that way of feeling the presence of the vastness of an unfamiliar world.

Appendix 1: Comparison and Causation

Inevitably, to speak of traditional Chinese medicine in English is to compare philosophies, cultures, and medical systems. Although in this book I have frequently considered together the practical and theoretical problems that occur in any modern medical context (and TCM certainly is a modern medicine), I concur with most writers on the history of Chinese medicine in their belief that profound differences persist between "Chinese" and "Western" (bio)medicine. Learning about TCM demands from us in "the West" an openness to concepts and facts that do not accord with many of our tacit assumptions about how the world works. One of those assumptions, for those of us who speak and think in languages allied to European civilization, is that events are caused by prior events.

Illness events are scary and uncomfortable, even for medical experts. A certain anxiety thus underlies our learning about a healing system that might compete, in a modern public health system, with the medical technologies on which we rely for our physical comfort, at times for our very life.[1] In making comparisons, we deploy a great many assumptions about what a medicine is or must be, and we presume we know what the "Western" medicine with which we are most familiar naturally and necessarily does. One commonsense truth you might recognize is, doctors are likely to know the cause of what ails us, and they are often able to eliminate that malignant thing. A cause and effect chain is interrupted by the doctor's medicines. Disease is eliminated when medical action attacks its causes.[2]

Thus when we compare medical systems, it seems to be imperative to address the question of cause. Historians have pointed out that in the

Western Hemisphere, ethers, witches, transgressions against God, and humoral excesses, seen as causes, have been at times as persuasive as are microbes, tumors, and genetic codes in our own time. Anthropology at first was a little naïve about translating the concept of cause, asking, for example, "What is 'the native's' equivalent of germs?" and answering this question with reports of superstitious "beliefs." Recent historical and anthropological research has been more open to cultural difference, seeking to understand holistically how people have answered the question "Why do we fall ill?"[3] The slight surprise is, not everyone has sought to answer this question by identifying a "cause" that would be recognizable, even in translation, to a biomedical practitioner.

E. E. Evans-Pritchard, for example, found rationality and practicality in Azande "mystical" explanations for specific afflictions: he made the answers to the questions of sufferers, "Why me? Why now?," a major topic for cultural and medical anthropology.[4] Geoffrey Lloyd has argued, in an important comparative project undertaken with historian of Chinese science Nathan Sivin, that "cause" is not a universal interest of philosophy or even science. It was, rather, a particular, and particularly influential, obsession of Platonic and Aristotelian disputation, yielding Aristotle's famous classification of causes (as if they were natural, and naturally distinct, things or entities for thought to act upon): material, formal, final, and efficient.[5] Modern medicine has mostly concerned itself with efficient or proximate causes, keying its therapeutics to the eradication of the single agent that is deemed to be the cause, in a linear sequence of events, of the disease. (Think viruses and bacteria, lesions and tumors, and lately, molecular genetics.) And in the many cases where cause is not definitively known, and therapies are not entirely successful at eliminating "the" cause, a pragmatist approach still talks in causal terms. We often resort, for example, to blaming "stress" for bringing on bouts of illness despite the notorious fuzziness of that concept.[6]

This contingent "Western" obsession with knowing and intervening in a linear process of causation at times has led some writers on Chinese medicine to assert that "Chinese thought is uninterested in cause."[7] This rather global remark would seem a little overconfident about the vastness that is "Chinese thought," but Ted Kaptchuk, its author, helpfully qualifies the idea in more historically specific ways. For example, in one of his many explicitly comparative moments, he gestures toward Aristotle:

> The idea of causation, central to Western thinking, is almost entirely absent [from Chinese thought and culture]. Aristotle . . . in his *Physics* . . . pens the archetypal formulation of this Western notion: "Men do not think they know a thing till they have grasped the 'why' of it (which is to grasp its primary cause)." For the Chinese, however, . . . there is no great need to search for a cause.[8]

No great need perhaps, but note that Nathan Sivin also deals, somewhat reluctantly, with the question of cause in Chinese medicine: "Although the three-type etiology [of inner, outer, and neither inner nor outer causes] was influential, discussions of causation were not very important either in basic or clinical medicine, far less important than accounts of the courses of disorders."[9] This nice distinction between *causes* and *courses* of disorders is a pithy summary of a key cultural difference. When, more than a decade later, Sivin engaged in a full-scale comparison between Chinese and Western medicine, his co-author Geoffrey Lloyd unpacked the Greek interest in causes, while in the Chinese sections of *The Way and the Word* Sivin analyzed ways of thinking not about causes but about courses of pathological events.[10]

In my own field research, I have noted that in the everyday life of clinical medicine today in China, doctors tend to be incurious about cause, a notion usually translated as *bingyin* (病因). Some hospital charts provide space for naming the *bingyin*, but quite often in practice it is left blank. Contemporary clinicians prefer to think in terms of pathology and physiology. These two modern terms are translated into Chinese as the patterns of appearance of illness and of life, *binglixue* (病理学) and *shenglixue* (生理学), respectively. Chinese medical doctors are more interested in course, in other words, than in cause.[11]

But let's talk about *bingyin*. Sivin shows that this is an old notion, and that even the classification of *bingyin* as "inner, outer, and neither inner nor outer causes" has a long pedigree.[12] He tends to translate *bingyin* as "causes," but he also subsumes the question of cause under more general considerations of etiology, showing that the process of disease appearance and development can be thought about apart from efforts to identify a determining cause. Yet because most of Sivin's pioneering 1987 study was an annotated translation of a basic TCM textbook published in 1972, he included and discussed the separate chapter of this modern work that was devoted to "causes of medical disorders."

Ted Kaptchuk, too, writing as an Asia-trained TCM physician as well as an inspired teacher and polemicist about Chinese medicine for Americans, has a chapter on "origins of disharmony" (though he subtitles it "or when a cause is not a cause"), using this term to cover the material a textbook would classify as *bingyin*. In my own work, I have translated *bingyin* as "illness factors" and followed the lead of other scholars in presenting illness factors as only one of many ways of understanding pathological process, or etiology. Once the event of illness is acknowledged to be the resultant of many overlapping processes both internal and external to bodies, the logical status of "the cause" in practical explanations and interventions is changed. Cause is no longer the master key that allows us to "grasp the 'why' of it." Indeed, a medicine that attends more to courses than causes will be especially interested in the "how" of it. And that process in which cause and effect are not distinguishable is what most of this book is about.[13]

Here's how a perfectly conventional (if slightly dated) textbook of TCM fundamentals opens its section on *bingyin*:

Chapter Four: Illness Factors, Illness Mechanisms

Chinese medicine holds that the connections among the various visceral systems of the body as well as between the human body and its environment are a process of both opposition and unity, unceasingly producing contradictions as well as resolving contradictions, and in this way maintaining a relative homeostatic balance (*dongtai pingheng* 动态平衡) which thereby safeguards the body's normal physiological activity. But for various reasons (*yin mouzhong yuanyin* 因某种原因), this relative homeostasis encounters damage, and when it cannot establish a spontaneous adjustment and recovery, the body can fall ill.[14]

This introductory language is showing its age, having been published in 1978 before the Marxist rhetoric derived from Mao's writings had declined in popularity. It is no longer necessary to see physiology as an instance of the dialectic using terms borrowed from Hegel, Marx, Engels, and Mao. But the dialectical logic of yin and yang, in their simultaneous opposition and unity, remains important in medicine. The yinyang dialectic makes "contradictions" such as causes and effects highly contingent, their identification dependent on the point when we intervene in the development of a pathology.[15] The notion of homeostatic balance, moreover, is a modern convenience, stepping in for the more ambiguous, not very scientific-sounding idea of "harmony" (*he* 和), which is much emphasized by more traditionalist contemporary writers who draw on classic philosophy to identify the underlying principles of TCM.[16]

The 1978 textbook's definitional opening continues:

The causes (*yuanyin* 原因) that damage the relatively homeostatic condition of the human body to induce disease are the bingyin, the illness factors. Our country's laboring people and the medical experts who passed through long periods of therapeutic practice know well that the factors that induce illness are many and various: untoward weather, contagious pestilences, emotional stimuli, bad diet and fatigue, extreme rage, external injuries from falls and knives, and even bugs and animals, all can do harm. Beyond this it is also known, in the disease course, causes and effects work both ways (*xianghu zuoyong* 相互作用), there are effect-things (*jieguode dongxi* 结果的东西) in each phase of disease which in another phase might become causes. Examples are phlegmy buildup, blood stasis, internal dampness, and inward fire; these are a loss of regularity in visceral systems, qi, and blood, which have formed as pathological products. Conversely, they can become factors (*bingbian de yinsu* 病变的因素) that in turn create certain pathological changes.

The paragraph that follows turns to the more important theme of the chapter, disease mechanism (*bingji* 病机) and pathological course (*bingli* 病理, lit. patterns of appearance of illness). Pointing out that all the many diseases have their own myriad symptomatic expressions, the text nevertheless assures us that there are "regular principles" underlying the patterns of disease manifestation, making it possible to understand the many factors in play in pathology. Wang Bing in the eighth century indicated the tactical importance of seeing some simpler underlying principles: "If you grasp the essentials of its mechanism, [he said] you will be able to either tweak minor problems or alter major ones, either work with the surface or be effective in depth."

These comments seem to make causes dependent on a rather holistic approach to pathological process. They are followed by a section entitled "Falling Ill," which one might think would lead us back to that prior event that causes disease to emerge. But the textbook authors insist on process over singular event nevertheless:

The occurrence of disease can be reduced to one point: It is none other than some degree of injury to the body's normal physiological activity. Under normal conditions, the [healthy] physiological activities of the human body are in a situation of relative homeostasis that is both opposed and unified, this is the so-called "yin even, yang hidden" (*yin ping yang mi* 阴平阳秘) state [referred to in the *Inner Canon*]. Under the function of an illness-inducing factor, the relative homeostasis of the body can be assaulted, i.e., "yin and yang lose attunement" (*yinyang shi tiao* 阴阳失调), and this is the beginning of disease.

We then turn to a technical aspect of this holistic argument: the "relative homeostasis" that needs to be safeguarded boils down to a relationship between normal qi (正气) and pathogenic qi (邪气); if normal qi is compromised in some way, it is much more likely that heteropathies will disrupt the proper balance of bodily processes. In the end, we are instructed:

> The occurrence and development of disease is simply the response to the struggle between normal and pathogenic qi under particular conditions. . . . The strength or weakness of normal qi mainly depends on constitutional factors, mental state, life environment and nutrition, exercise, etc.

In its attempts to define and mobilize "cause" for clinical attention, this textbook does not admit reductionism: "falling ill" is the result of many illness factors interacting "under particular conditions." And even these conditions can look a lot like illness-inducing factors. In what follows one learns that "mental state" is closely related to the seven emotional excesses (*qiqing* 七情), "environment" contains the six climatic "pernicious influences" (*liuying* 六淫), diet can introduce toxins (*du* 毒), and so on.

When it comes to designing a therapeutic intervention, it is clear that TCM actors cannot attack a single chief cause, conventionally identified, of the complaints they must treat. How, then, do they decide on an intervention, when there are so many strands of influence in play? How do they, following Wang Bing, "grasp the essentials of its mechanism, . . . either tweak minor problems or alter major ones, either work with the surface or be effective in depth"? Even if they refuse the idea of disease causes altogether, surely they want to be able to *cause* an improvement in the patient's condition. Right?

Chapter 4 of this book has sought to answer these questions, especially using the language of "nudging" processes of flow and transformation in desired directions. Insofar as my arguments concerning "things, thought, and action" have successfully characterized a complex form of agency and efficacy for "traditional" medicine in China, we have been returned to the question of efficacy itself.[17] Bearing in mind that Chinese herbal medicine, acupuncture, and massage are markedly effective for controlling a "myriad" of symptoms, perhaps a sympathetic reflection on some philosophical dilemmas in TCM can invite us to reconsider not only causation but even the forms of action and efficacy we find collectively desirable in many domains of action. Healing does not require mastery of a linear cause and effect mechanism—all clinicians really know this, actually, biomedical reductionism notwithstanding—nor does it have to engage in a half-controlled series of billiard ball "efficient causes" pushing discrete things around.

Chinese medicine seeks efficacy in a different way. One only needs to reflect on any common herbal prescription: this classic gathering of complexities, each component a natural thing known to mobilize a set of characters and flavors, with each thing also having propensities for affecting particular bodily systems, is a polymorphous agency. An herbal prescription addresses and counters every symptomatic chain of events, touches every discomfort and worry brought by the sufferer, in its mixture, weaving a responsive web of powers that can be applied to the disorder like a well-tailored garment of care. This is not a romanticized replacement for a hard-headed medicine of cause and effect. Rather, it is the kind of action understood and undertaken in an everyday way by those who use traditional Chinese medicine.

Appendix 2: Yes, Medicine Is Thought!

I met Zhang Dong in the summer of 2018 during a one-month stay in Beijing. Dr. Zhang, at the request of our mutual friend Lai Lili, agreed to host a University of Chicago student intern in his clinics in a hospital that is part of the China Academy of Chinese Medical Sciences network. Dr. Lai, the intern Alex Ding, and I had one interesting planning meeting with him, then Alex was able to spend some fruitful afternoons observing, as a medical anthropologist, his practice. Dr. Zhang gave us copies of his recent book *Original Qi, Vital Machine.*[1] Eventually, after I had left Beijing, he was able to have more relaxed conversations with Lili and Alex. On these sociable occasions, which I hope will continue when I am in Beijing, Zhang Dong confessed that he originally had no interest in Chinese medicine, hoping instead to read and write philosophy. He especially appreciated ancient metaphysics (both "Eastern" and "Western" varieties), and he was also much attracted to Nietzschean thought. (In the preface translated here, he cites Karl Jaspers, a Nietzsche scholar.)

I began to read Dr. Zhang's book at a time when I was revising my Terry Lectures into book form. His interests, both clinical and philosophical, impressed me as being very similar to my own, while at the same time being nearly untranslatable into Anglophone scholarship. As I simultaneously read his book and wrote my own, I found some of his views extraordinarily confirming of things I thought I knew about Chinese medicine. Zhang does not so much describe the current state of practice in TCM as advocate for a broad and difficult evolution toward a better state of play, and toward a greater influence for TCM on world values. And he does so as a clinician, that is, as an actor who thinks like a pragmatist to grapple with demanding things.

The structure of Zhang's book makes his commitment to Chinese medical things, thought, and action clear. Dr. Zhang devotes the first section of *Original Qi, Vital Machine* to a full discussion of several classic herbal prescriptions and his particular modifications of them. This technical section is followed by a number of case reports from his clinical work, meant to demonstrate both the action of the formulas and the responsiveness of his clinical thinking to the transformations of the myriad things. The latter part of the book contains chapters on "The *Dao De Jing* and Chinese Medicine," "The *Book of Changes* and Chinese Medicine," and "The Way and Practical Arts." Attaching case reports from three of his students in a last chapter, he then concludes with a comparative afterword.

In my own writing I found it convenient to make frequent reference to Zhang Dong's arguments, so I decided to append this translation of his book's fascinating preface. As I noted above, his thought is hard to translate. It is complex, sometimes technical, and thoroughly situated in long-standing debates and speculations that have appeared only in Chinese. Here I have translated, as closely and literally as possible, only the preface of *Original Qi, Vital Machine*, and I have not tried to explain the many mysteries that will likely frustrate readers in English. As we read theorists of TCM, I think we have to take Zhang Dong's own advice about the challenge posed by the classical Chinese language of philosophy: "If you reflect often on the puzzle these words present, the meaning might come on its own."

Zhang Dong, *Original Qi, Vital Machine*

PREFACE

On the Title of This Book

Without doubt, Chinese medicine's most important classic is the *Yellow Emperor's Inner Canon* (*Huangdi Nei Jing* 黄帝内经; hereafter, *Inner Canon*). The *Inner Canon* includes two books, the "Plain Questions" (*Suwen* 素问) and the "Divine Pivot" (*Lingshu* 灵枢). Quan Yuanqi (sixth century CE), in the earliest commentary on the *Suwen* states that "*su*" [plain, simple] is equivalent to "*ben*" (本 root). So the "Plain Questions" thus amounts to questions and answers concerning original root sources. *Su* is also equivalent to *pu* (朴) or simple. The *Shuowen* (a second-century dictionary) notes that *pu* refers to the plainness of wood (*mu su* 木素). In the nineteenth chapter of the *Dao De Jing* we find: "Look for the basic (*su*), embrace the simple (*pu*), lessen self-interest, starve desire." In the *Dao De Jing*, "the simple" is another word for the Way (*dao*). According to the *Dao De Jing*, "The oscillation of the Way, this is what is called simple. Although it is a small thing, nothing under heaven could be bigger." In the text that follows, we see, "The One—this is the origin; that is, original qi (*yuanqi* 元气)." Thus it is that the "Plain Questions" is an interrogation of the Way and of the origin in the realm of medicine. This is why this book is called "Original Qi," expressing its intention of exploring and interrogating origin qi through medicine.

In the "Divine Pivot," or the *Lingshu*, "*ling*" means divinely vital [sacred (*shen* 神)], and "*shu*" is equivalent to mechanism [machine, or works, or what turns like a hinge]. So *lingshu* is equivalent to "vital machine," or *shenji* (神机). The *Transmitted Changes* states, "Isn't knowing the machine [a way to know] its divine vitality? . . . The machine is the most minuscule action, the moment when you can first see [a tendency toward] good or evil [events]. The lord acts as soon as he sees the mechanism turning, he doesn't wait for the day of the outcome." In the *Zhuangzi* we read, "The myriad things all come out from the works, and all return to the works." This machine (or works) can channel divine vitality, that's why it's called vital. The *Transmitted Changes* says, "The unfathomable in the yinyang process, this is called *shen*-vitality." What is unfathomable in yinyang is the changes (*bianhua* 变化) of origin qi.

It follows that the "Plain Questions" and the "Divine Pivot" are in effect one book that came out under two titles, like the *Dao De Jing*, in which "*Dao*" (the Way) and "*De*" (virtue/power) come out paired, though they are different terms. The Way is the base (*ti* 体) and virtue is its application (*yong* 用). The Way is the root and basis, and virtue is the Way put to use.

Similarly, in the *Inner Canon*, the "Plain Questions" is the basis and the "Divine Pivot" is the application. And this present book is one base and one use: original qi is the base and the vital machine is the application.

"Exploring the Way of Pre-Qin Medicine" is also in the title. Pre-Qin refers to all the historical periods prior to the founding of the Qin Dynasty in 221 BCE, namely, the Xia, Shang, and Western Zhou Dynasties, and the Spring and Autumn and Warring States Periods. Pre-Qin thought and culture is the fountainhead of Chinese culture, and has deeply influenced Chinese people's thinking. The Pre-Qin Period produced the *Book of Changes* [hereafter, the *Changes*] and the representative works that are pinnacles of the culture of the Spring and Autumn Period and the Warring States Period.

German philosopher Karl Jaspers famously called this long historical epoch the "axial age"; the period that controlled, guided, and motivated the meaning of all human culture. This period was a crucial breakthrough time for the spirit of human civilization. In the axial age, every civilization produced great spiritual teachers: Socrates, Plato, Sakyamuni, Confucius, Laozi, each of them a founder of his own thought system, who together forged the spiritual foundation for humankind's civilizations. Even up to the present, humans are still standing on this foundation. Jaspers also wrote, "Up to the present day, humanity has relied for its existence on everything that the axial age produced, contemplated, and created. Every new leap [in thought] recalls this era in order to reignite the flame. It has ever been thus. The axial age has been the universal spiritual force opening all the potentials for cultural awakening, renewal, and return."

The Book of Changes and other cosmological works are all classics of this generative period. Mr. Huang Moya has said that the Pre-Qin was the head of Chinese culture, and scholars agree that this has properly been called our cultural golden age. This era produced Chinese medicine, along with legendary doctors like Bian Que, Yi He, and Yi Huan. This era's thought is thus the source of the thought of the *Inner Canon*.

For a long time now, people have been asking, the times have so clearly progressed and developed, why did China's forebears venerate the past?

YES, MEDICINE IS THOUGHT!

Take Chinese medicine as an example: the *Inner Canon* and the *Treatise on Cold Disorders* are not just ordinary Chinese medical classics, they are simply the unsurpassable high points of medicine, and they have been wellsprings of medical thought (*yixue sixiang* 医学思想) for the ages. This has a very close relationship with China's traditional modes of thought. As I discuss in the afterword, the essential difference between Chinese medicine and Western medicine is not what drugs are used, nor is it a matter of injections versus acupuncture. Rather, it is the difference between two modes of thought. The West holds that the natural method is the epistemology of a subject-object divide (*wuwo fenli* 物我分离 [lit. separation between self and object]), but the Chinese ancients' way of understanding nature is to consciously adopt a non-dualist epistemology in which subject and object are unified (*wuwo heyi* 物我合一).

This [ancient epistemology] demands a consciousness and a kind of action that is unthinking, unmoving, non-desiring. Indeed, it is just as the *Transmitted Changes* says: "The Changes are the unthought, they are spontaneous, not deliberate action. They are still and unmoving, yet they respond in accord with all the lesser causes passing through the world. As for things not intended by the mind of the world (*tianxia zhi shen* 天下之神), when we ask 'who did it,' the answer lies here." From this we can see, only if there is "responsiveness with all the causes passing through the world" can nature (*ziran* 自然) truly be comprehended. And with regard to "things not intended by the mind of the world, when we ask who did it," this means that only a few sages can really understand in this way successfully. Moreover, one would need a peaceful natural environment. Though conditions of life were far from perfect in ancient times, and were materially lacking, they certainly achieved a life environment of peacefulness, naturalness, and non-desiring. Though people could not seek much help from external things, they could more naturally reflect inward on their own heart-mind and body-self. A few people, such as Fu Xi, Zhou Gong, Laozi, Zhuangzi, and so on, were able to make the self/mind and nature correspond (相应), achieving a direct knowledge of nature's aims. Their way of knowing nature was rather different from the objectivist/dualist methods of the West, and as material conditions developed, this kind of epistemology of the ancients came to be more and more unknown to and unable to be used by people of later times. The dualist (*wuwo fenlide* 物我分离的) epistemology of later times gradually became the mainstream. Although this approach developed quite rapidly, its very nature was quite limited and partial, and it made it impossible for later generations to know or experience the [ancient] epistemology that draws subject and object together. But for us this kind of knowledge of nature is deeply rooted (*benrande* 本然的), there's no substitute for it: this is one of the main reasons later generations have revered the ancients.

Though we cannot fully recover that past, fortunately the sages of old left writings and literatures for their descendants. We should do as Zhang Zhongjing recommended, "Diligently seek lessons from the past"—we should especially seek out Pre-Qin Chinese medicine, against the background of Pre-Qin culture, because that era is the source of Chinese medicine.

If the *Inner Canon* is the source of Chinese medicine for later generations, even more is the medicine of Pre-Qin times the source for the *Inner Canon*. But the medical knowledge of the Pre-Qin Periods has not come down to us, how can we seek it out? Fortunately, the ancients told us that the patterns of the myriad things all pass through each other (*wanwu zhi li shi xiangtongde* 万物之理是相通的), so if we are just versed in the worldview and thought style of the ancients, there will be traces we can follow. Pre-Qin Chinese medicine is born from the cultural background of Pre-Qin culture, its view of the human body is necessarily convergent with (*xiangtongde* 相通的) its views on dealing with natural phenomena, because the ancients held that heaven and the human are mutually responsive. Thus, the literature of the Pre-Qin eras, all the various authors, the Huang-Lao scholars, astronomical calendrics, even oracle bone writings and the discoveries of the evidentiary school and so forth, all are important literatures we should study. In doing so, we trace back to the sources, seeking the roots of Chinese medicine.

The great Confucian scholar of the Northern Song, Zhang Zai, uttered a famous parallelism: "Establish mind for the universe, establish life for the people, thoroughly continue to study the sages, and thus inaugurate true peace for all the ages." Tracing Pre-Qin culture back to its sources, exploring the Way of Pre-Qin medicine, is a way of learning from the august sages. This is the duty of everyone inclined toward the field of Chinese medicine.

Starting Points   The *Inner Canon* is the classic of classics in Chinese medicine, and throughout history every medical expert and every school has taken the *Inner Canon* as its ancestor. The medical sage Zhang Zhongjing in the *Treatise on Cold Disorders (Shang Han Lun* 伤寒论*)* noted that in his writing he had consulted the nine scrolls of the "Plain Questions." But where did the *Inner Canon* come from? Why would one even ask such a question? Because the *Inner Canon* presents us with many "whys." For example, what is the reasoning involved in "pairing" the five yin viscera (*zang* 脏) with the six yang viscera (*fu* 腑)? It would be okay to pair five yin viscera with five yang viscera, so why would [the sixth *fu*] the "triple burner" be added? The triple burner has a name but no discrete form (*xing* 形). When later a "pericardium" (*xinbao* 心包) is added to match the triple burner, what's the real significance of this? We also know that the mature yang (*taiyang* 太阳) circulation channel is triple yang, yang qi at its most energetic, so why would it be matched to winter and the water phase? Is this a way of counter-matching yang? So, why then is the mature yin (*taiyin* 太阴) channel paired with damp and the earth phase? Taiyin is triple yin, and damp and earth both also belong to yin. These kinds of questions are all needed to answer the bigger question, what is the general logic of pairing the visceral systems? What is the logic of matching the twelve channels [to other functional correlates]? Another example: according to the *Inner Canon*, "When the liver reaches severe pendulousness (*gan zhi xuanjue* 肝至悬绝), death will occur in eighteen days." Why? If you don't understand the background and sources of the *Inner Canon*, such questions are very hard to resolve. Most who have researched the *Inner Canon* dwell on what the text says, then they simply do as it says. But very few have explored the question of why the *Inner Canon* was written in the way it was, what is the logic of what is written? What is the real meaning of what is written?

Apart from these considerations, what is the deeper significance of exploring the background logic of the *Inner Canon*? We know that the *Inner Canon* is a major source of the medical thought that came after it, but the *Inner Canon* is not a complete work covering the medical knowledge that preceded it. Perhaps it is only a small part of that precursor medicine. And if that small part operated such a great influence on later generations, well, couldn't the lost thought of the *Inner Canon*'s precursor medicine—for example, the medical thought of Bian Que or Cang Gong—possibly have an even deeper and greater influence? Today, these forms of medical thought have been lost to us and we seem to have no way of recovering them. But these lost forms of medical thought and the *Inner Canon* have the same earlier sources. If we understand the origins of the thought of the *Inner Canon*, then we have found the thread leading us back to the thought of these earlier medical thinkers. If you don't understand the sources of the thought in the *Inner Canon*, then you are only able to passively follow its directions without understanding why you are doing that. You would "know how things are done without knowing why." There would be no way to truly comprehend the implicit significance of the *Inner Canon*, nor would it be possible to act well. At the same time, if you cannot truly understand the essence of the theory of Chinese medicine, there's no way you can satisfactorily critique it. You can only have a personal opinion. For example, there are those who say that the five phases [system of analysis] is useless trash, but if Chinese medicine discards [*Inner Canon* knowledge] of this kind then it becomes a spring without water or a tree without roots.

An example is research on the channels. If you don't understand what the ancients said about the nature of the channels, then you cannot work out a rigorous approach to research. And if your research approaches are all wrong, how can you get results? For example, in the *Inner Canon* it says that the visceral systems and the nine orifices are all connected. There are many

scholars who try to use the methods of modern medicine to find the [ana-
tomical] basis of this [holism], following the nerves and blood vessels, or
studying hormones, embryology, and molecular biology to find evidence. Is
this way of thinking correct? The *Inner Canon* also says that the nine orifices
and the nine regions [of China] are connected, but it's hard to imagine that
you could find a biophysical relationship between the nine orifices and the
nine regions. This just shows that these researchers do not grasp the true
meaning of what the ancients were saying. If we are not clear on the basic
meaning of these ancient sentences, how can we do research on them? What
is the point of doing research on imaginary things?

For some years now I've been doing research that traces Chinese medicine, and especially the *Inner Canon*, back to its root sources in Chinese
thought. There's no doubt that the thought of the *Inner Canon* is similar
to that of its sources in [Pre-Qin] times; but what are the sources of this
early thought itself? Chinese medicine did not just spring into existence in
one leap, with the *Inner Canon*. It slowly accumulated, it was gathered over
a long period from culture, theory, and experience. But one point we can
admit: the *Inner Canon* was deeply influenced by Pre-Qin thought and culture, so no research on the sources of the *Inner Canon* can evade or bypass its
context (*beijing* 背景) in Pre-Qin culture. We can also see in the scholarship
that the *Inner Canon* was not the only form of medical thought that developed in the context of Pre-Qin culture. There were many other scholarly
currents and styles of thought that possibly were lost to us early on. These
early forms of medical thought may be partly hidden within the Pre-Qin
classics and the *Inner Canon*; this is what the present work wants to focus on.

As can be seen from the title of the *Yellow Emperor's Inner Canon*, the
soil that originated and developed Chinese medicine is traditional Chinese
culture. Traditional Chinese culture takes Confucianism, Buddhism, and
Daoism as representative. Confucianism and Daoism are indigenous forms
of thought and culture, though Buddhist culture is not. Daoist thought
and culture takes the *Dao De Jing* of Laozi as its primary canon and the
wellspring of its thought; the canon of Confucianism is the *Six Classics*.

Confucius, the founder of China's Confucian current, late in his life edited the *Book of Songs* (*shijing* 诗经), the *Book of History* (*shujing* 书经), the *Classic of Rites* (*liji* 礼记), the *Book of Changes* (*yijing* 易经), the *Book of Music* (*yuejing* 乐经), and the *Spring and Autumn Annals* (*chunqiu* 春秋); later people called these the Six Classics, but the *Changes* is positioned as the head of the six. It is the classic of classics for Confucian thought. Daoism emphasizes non-action and departure from the worldly, while Confucianism engages the world with its "doctrine of the mean." Both of these types of thought deeply influenced the *Inner Canon* and the later development of Chinese medicine.

As can be seen from its title, *Yellow Emperor's Inner Canon,* there is a deep connection between the so-called Yellow Emperor and the Daoist thought of Laozi. The ancients of China spoke of the union of Laozi's and the Yellow Sovereign's thought as the "Huang Lao School," a current of thought that began in the Warring States Period and extended into the time of the Western Han. In the *Historical Records* Sima Qian repeatedly mentions the Huang Lao School, and the *Inner Canon* is one of its texts.

The thinking of the *Inner Canon* is quite continuous with the thought of Laozi. For example, we know that "non-action" is one of the core ideas of the *Dao De Jing*. See the *Dao De Jing*: "It is the sage who sets up affairs for non-action, he acts but does not preach it with words." "The Way is non-acting but it is never inactive." And then see the "Plain Questions" (*juan* 5), "It is the sage who does things as non-action, he can rest in absolute stillness, and desireless can enter the space of vacuity."

The plain and simple (*pu* 朴) is also a key concept in the *Dao De Jing*. See, for example, "The Way is often vacant, this is called plain, although it is a small thing, there is nothing under heaven that could be more vast." "Food that is sweet, clothes that are beautiful, a peaceful house, routines you enjoy—if the ruler's vision is the same and they hear the same cock crow, the people will live to a ripe old age and will not restlessly move about." The "Plain Questions" (*juan* 1) similarly states: "Food that is beautiful, clothes that are proper, enjoyable routines, accord between the lowly and the highly placed: such a people is called plain."

The *Dao De Jing* strongly emphasizes the "One": "Heaven achieves Oneness so as to be clear, earth achieves Oneness so as to be solid, spirit/ vitality achieves Oneness so as to be magical (*ling* 灵), grains achieve Oneness so as to flourish; the ruler achieves Oneness so as to order (*zheng* 正) all under heaven." The "Plain Questions" (*juan* 19) has a similar message: "Governing and regulating deviations and adjustments, this Way lies with the One." We can see here that the *Dao De Jing* is one of the thought wellsprings that produced the *Inner Canon,* and that the *Inner Canon* inherited and continued the thought of the Daoists.

The Pre-Qin Period had already produced a rich body of life-nurturing (*yangsheng* 养生) thought, an example being the *Moving Qi Inscriptions* (*xingqi yupeiming* 行气玉佩铭), a work that is verified to be of the late Warring States Period [fourth century BCE]. This is one of our country's first extant works of cultural materials on Qigong theory.

The *Moving Qi Inscriptions* states: "To circulate qi [i.e., breath], breathe deeply so it accumulates. Accumulated, it can expand, when it expands it can descend [in the body]. When it has reached a low place, fix it. When it is fixed in place, hold it steady. Once it is steady it will become like a sprouting plant, and sprouted it will grow. As it grows, it will retrace its path. Retracing its path, it reaches toward heaven. Heaven's machine throbs above, earth's machine throbs below. If you follow this, you live; if you oppose it, you die."[2]

In the *Zhuangzi* one finds many traces of Daoist life-nurturing (*yangsheng* 养生) thought. Yangsheng thought from the Pre-Qin was later passed down as alchemical Daoism, forming into a unique life-view. This kind of knowledge came down to us not only as the study of Huang Lao, but it also developed into a completely alchemical yangsheng system. You could say that this system was directly transmitted from the Pre-Qin Daoist masters and that it made an important contribution to medicine, health, and life-nurturing. And you could also say that it forms one unified set of yangsheng methods with the medical system inherited from the *Inner Canon,* and it can be used to treat diseases. Unfortunately, historically this unique system of thought was only transmitted secretly among Daoist alchemists.

The *Book of Changes* was earlier than the *Dao De Jing*, and its form of thought also deeply influenced the *Inner Canon;* it was a very important source of the thought system (*tixi* 体系) of the *Inner Canon.*

The *Yellow Emperor's Inner Canon* and the Daoists' alchemical life-nurturance approach continued the thought of Laozi and Zhuangzi and that of the *Book of Changes,* but the two currents later took divergent directions of development. The medicine that followed upon the *Inner Canon* took as its main guide the *Dao De Jing's* principle "The Three gives birth to the myriad" and the *Changes'* dictum "The latter heaven acts in accord with the seasons of heaven," thus developing a latter heaven-oriented [i.e., empirical and experiential] medicine system. But the Daoist alchemical life-nurturing tradition developed with Daoism's mantra "embrace the origin and preserve unity," and with the idea from the *Changes* that the former heaven [the innate] never goes against heaven's patterns (*tianshi* 天时), later developing a former heaven-oriented medical system. These two strains can stand side by side to be called the two pillars of China's traditional medicine. But because the aims of the two medical systems differ in their historical factors, one is quite prominent in the world and the other is hidden within the world, there are rather few who can discern the latter, hidden tradition.

This book takes the *Dao De Jing* and the *Book of Changes* as its ancestors, tracing back the thought sources in the time of the *Inner Canon,* penetrating the life-nurturing thought of the Daoists, working out thereby a "new" medical way of thinking, and showing it in use in clinical practice. This so-called novelty is perhaps even more ancient than TCM, because it comes from the time before the *Inner Canon* was compiled. The production of this kind of medical thought is perhaps a matter of the channel forming only when the water arrives. It's just that a great deal was lost and now can be found "anew." In this book, everyone can gradually come to realize that if you want to learn Chinese medicine, you must understand China's traditional culture, understand the style of thought of China's ancients: this is an essential prerequisite, there's no other way.

I need to explain, for the sake of readers who don't read classical Chinese, in this book the classical language is sometimes translated into modern vernacular Chinese, but there are still sentences remaining that will be difficult. Especially the *Dao De Jing* is very poetic; if you don't leave it in its classical form, its meaning and flavor are quite changed. If you try to translate one word and phrase at a time, rather than getting a sense of the whole message, you can skew its basic meaning or just miss the forest for seeing the trees. Therefore, in the translations into modern Chinese that I have used, I have sometimes simply not translated, leaving some difficult words in their untranslated context. I hope readers will read these closely, like poems, and read them again and again. If you reflect often on the puzzle they present, the meaning might come on its own.

Furthermore, this book adopted a "flashback" (*daoxu* 倒叙) method, a kind of retrospective narration, first writing out the drug formulas and cases [and then taking up some philosophical ideas]. The reader who finds the way back to the source naturally can perceive the theories and regularities [in these myriad clinical details].

Essential Meanings   This book takes its nourishment from the three classic works: the *Dao De Jing*, the *Book of Changes*, and the *Yellow Emperor's Inner Canon*. The *Dao De Jing* and the *Changes* take up the patterns (*li* 理) of heaven and earth, with the Way of the human body also included. The *Inner Canon* says, "The transformations cannot be replaced, the timing cannot be opposed." This is *Dao De Jing* thought: "Assiduously guard its qi, don't make it deviate [far from its natural path]. It is necessary to nurture and to harmonize, address its comings and goings." This is also *Changes* thought, and the author is thoroughly in accord with this aim, hence this book.

One of the core concepts of the *Dao De Jing* is non-action, and the root of treating illness ought to be allowing the original qi of the body to heal without action. Modern medicine takes disease as its center, it seeks out the disease and actively eradicates it. But the viewpoint of this book is, when the human body shifts from ill-health to health, it results from a process in which origin qi moves from injury to recovery. Restoration of health is nothing other than the restoration of origin qi to its proper state of non-action. When origin qi is neither active nor inert, then and only then can the body be truly healthy. When health is restored, disease is naturally driven out. This is why Sunzi in *The Art of War* ("Attack by Stratagem," *juan* 3) says: "Hence to fight and conquer in all your battles is not supreme excellence; supreme excellence consists in breaking the enemy's resistance without fighting." Likewise, modern medicine never sees victory over disease in all its battles. The method in this book prefers not to deploy troops; rather than trying to attack disease, we like to see illness depart on its own.

The *Dao De Jing* and the *Book of Changes*, as well as the life-nurturing thought of the alchemical Daoists, have hidden within them the method of allowing original qi to recover its proper non-action. "The Way gives birth to the One, One gives birth to the Two, Two gives birth to Three, Three gives birth to the myriad things." The One here is original qi; "Two" is yin and yang; and bodily visceral systems, blood, and qi are examples of the myriad things of the human body. If you would make bodily original qi non-active, you need to make the body's "myriad things" return to the One. Only with a return to the One can original qi be restored to non-action. This is the process that the Daoists called the latter heaven returning to the former heaven. The *Changes* held that the key to the latter heaven returning to the former heaven was assignable to the "fu" graph and the "gou" graph, what Shao Yongcheng of the Song Period called "heaven's root" and "moon's cavity."

The movement of the body's visceral systems, blood, and qi is like the Taiji Diagram, in which yin and yang go up on the right and down on the left to make a circle. The rising on the left is yang, it gives birth and grows, and the falling on the left is yin, it collects and stores. The qi that births and grows and the qi that collects and stores "flow together and become a harmony" (*chongqi yiwei he* 冲气以为和), and their cooperation thus becomes the center of the circle. This process has two "works," or pivots. One is the yang starting point of qi transformation becoming a circular motion, that is to say, the starting point of birthing and growing qi; the Daoists called this "heaven's root," in response to the time of heaven [a two-week year segment called] winter's arrival, that point when one yang first appears. The other is the yin starting point of qi transformation becoming a circular motion, that is to say, the starting point of collecting and storing qi; the Daoists called this "moon cavity," in response to the time of heaven [called] summer's arrival, that point when one yin first appears. These two points, heaven's root and the moon cavity, are pivots of the human body's circular motion of qi transformation, and they are turning points of the origin qi of the latter heaven, they are crucial points.

The author takes his basis from these three points, the center, heaven's root, and the moon cavity, and takes the pattern of yin and yang returning to the one, to set up two formulas: Returning-to-the-One Liquor and Seeing Double Decoction.

Returning-to-the-One Liquor is born from Four Counters Decoction, it places aconite (*fuzi*, 附子 monkshood) in the major "ministerial" (*chen* 臣) position, according to the starting-to-move pivot as one yang turns toward birthing and growing, causing the qi of birth and growth to be renewed. Similarly, roasted licorice root (*zhigancao* 炙甘草) occupies the "courtier" drug (*jun* 君) position, making use of licorice's ability to smooth/harmonize the middle and induce birth-growth qi to return to the center; dried ginger links with the aconite and licorice root to be the assistant and emissary (*zuoshi* 佐使). This prescription is set up on the heaven's root and center turning points, it initiates the birthing and growing machine, and leads the qi of birth and growth and the qi of collection and storage to flow together and harmonize, bringing harmony to the center.

Seeing Double Decoction is born from Managing the Middle Pills (*lizhongwan* 理中丸). It takes red ginseng as the "monarch," in accord with summer's arrival of the one yin that stimulates the collecting and storing machine, leading the qi of storage and collection to renew itself. Similarly, roasted licorice root (*zhigancao* 炙甘草) occupies the "minister" drug position, making use of licorice's ability to smooth/harmonize the middle and induce collection and storage qi to return to the center. Dried ginger and baishu link with the ginseng and licorice root to be the "assistant" and "emissary" (*zuoshi* 佐使) drugs. This prescription is set up on the moon cavity turning point, it initiates the collecting and storing machine, and leads the qi of collection and storage and the qi of birth and growth to converge and harmonize, bringing harmony to the center.

The *Yellow Emperor's Inner Canon* says, "Assiduously guard its qi, don't force it to asymmetric change." These two formulas assiduously guard the yinyang machine, lead yin and yang to harmonize, allow original qi to spontaneously recover, such that original qi neither acts nor fails to act, such that one does not treat illness, yet illness departs of itself. The goal of these two formulas is to harmonize the qi of birthing and growing and the qi of collecting and storing, when yin and yang converge in harmony then original qi recovers, and when original qi is recovered then illness is banished.

The cases in this book come from the work of the author and his students. They include many sorts of diseases, and we have tried to avoid duplications.

This book attempts, through a deeper kind of excavation, to explore the sources of Chinese medicine in China's traditional culture and thus more effectively find out the living wellsprings of Chinese medicine. In this way we can make a new kind of thought that is rooted in the soil of traditional Chinese culture, and we can bring new life to Chinese medicine.

Notes

Chapter 1. Science, Civilization, and Practice

1. On changes taking place in the world of Chinese medical and scientific publishing in the early 1980s, see Farquhar, "Rewriting Traditional Medicine."

2. There are many reflections on the philosophy of biology in Needham's *Science and Civilisation in China*. In those pages, he often expressed his commitment to an organicist understanding of living systems, as opposed to a "Newtonian" reductionism. See, for example, Needham, *Science and Civilisation in China*, 2:291–93.

3. Sigerist, *Medicine and Human Welfare*; Mead, *Continuities in Cultural Evolution*; Geertz, *Islam Observed*; Douglas, *Thinking in Circles*; Lopez, *Scientific Buddha*; Doniger, *Against Dharma*; Ricoeur, *Freud and Philosophy*; Smith, *Natural Reflections*.

4. I think this interest prefigured Needham's turn to Chinese thought. Even etymologically, the idea of "morphogenesis" is eerily "Asian" and very consistent with some arguments derived from Chinese medicine and traditional Chinese sciences (see Nappi, *Monkey and the Inkpot*; Farquhar, "Objects, Processes, and Female Infertility"; Farquhar, "Multiplicity, Point of View, and Responsibility") and ancient Chinese metaphysical writings (see Zhuang, *Zhuangzi*).

5. Foucault, "Introduction" to Canguilhem, *Normal and the Pathological*.

6. Science and Technology Studies (STS) has turned to the history of "co-construction" in networks that include actors both human and non-human. See, e.g., Latour, *Pasteurization of France*; Latour, *Pandora's Hope*; Pickering, *Mangle of Practice*; Rheinberger, *Epistemology of the Concrete*; Daston, "Introduction" to *Biographies of Scientific Objects*; Mitchell, "Can the Mosquito Speak?" Anthropologist Casper Bruun Jensen has provided an excellent discussion of co-construction in his "New Ontologies?" The twentieth-century historians of science were more narrowly sociological in the sense that they were interested only in human knowledge and action.

7. Law, "One-World World?"

8. On ontological pluralism, see James, *Pluralistic Universe,* and Connolly, *Pluralism.*

9. This was certainly the case for astronomical cosmology, meteorology, some kinds of mathematics, and for a number of technical engineering fields like hydraulics and metallurgy, weaving and printing, and various forms of sophisticated manufacturing. See especially Needham, *Grand Titration.*

10. His symptoms of Parkinson's disease were by that time fairly advanced, though Needham was still actively guiding the research for *Science and Civilisation.* He appeared rarely at the NRI Library and seldom gave interviews; he died in 1995, outliving Lu Gwei-Djen by three or four years. Dr. Lu graciously agreed to talk to me, even though I was a very junior and short-term visitor.

11. On the notion of "currents" of science and history in China, see Scheid, *Currents of Tradition.* Ren Yingqiu adopted the idea of scholarly currents (*xuepai* 学派) to organize his important mid-twentieth-century work on the history of medicine in China, founding a series of medical college classes organized around the "teachings of the various [medical] specialists" (*gejia xueshuo* 各家学说).

12. There was one English-language history of medicine in China available at the time, that of Wong Chimin and Lien-teh Wu, *History of Chinese Medicine.* This book devoted most of its space to the recent development of biomedicine in China, and its single chapter on the history of Chinese medicine in China was not characterized by the high level of scholarship associated with the Needham and Lu project.

13. Lu and Needham, *Celestial Lancets.*

14. Hart, "On the Problem of Chinese Science"; Scheid and Virág, "Introduction to History of Science."

15. Let me finish the story of my meeting with Dr. Lu several decades ago. The planned sixth volume of *Science and Civilisation*—the one broadly covering the biological sciences, about which I was asking—has now appeared in the form of six monographs, all of them deriving from extensive collaboration with other China scholars who kept on working in the *Science and Civilisation* project long after Joseph Needham and Lu Gwei-Djen died in the 1990s. Volume 6, book number 1 on botany, the one with Dr. Lu's fingerprints most evident on it, appeared in 1986. The one that looks the most like a history of medicine is volume 6, number 6, assembled from Lu and Needham's occasional writings on the subject of medicine and edited by Nathan Sivin. Sivin handles the problem of translation rather differently

than Needham and Lu themselves did, and he discusses this difference, and his own historiographical commitments, in his excellent introduction to the monograph. He can be credited with having tackled the problem of translating Chinese medicine more head-on than most, and with his own very sensible system of terms. But he has not added to his copious writings on the history of science in China a comprehensive history of medicine in China.

16. One of my MD-PhD friends practicing in the US liked to state on his website that he "had a religious commitment to evidence-based medicine." From a patient's point of view, I could report numerous little instances of the magic and mysteries encountered and acknowledged in routine clinical work. Thanks for this insight are due to my kind and honest doctors in biomedical clinics over the years, and to Barry Saunders and Jens Foell, MD magicians par excellence.

17. Cf. Lloyd and Sivin, *Way and the Word*. In this explicitly comparative work, Sivin does count Chinese medicine among the sciences, although he refuses to use the abstract epistemological notion of science (in the singular) for any of the premodern Chinese knowledge-and-practice systems, even mathematics (page 227).

18. Kenneth Miller's website suggests that he might have been driven to this trope by creationist students challenging him in his evolutionary biology classes. On the "versus," see Smith, "Religion, Science, and the Humanities."

19. James, *Essays in Radical Empiricism*, 5–6.

20. On immunity, see Anderson and Mackay, *Intolerant Bodies*. On metabolism, see Landecker, "Metabolism, Autonomy, Individuality." On stress, see Young, "Discourse on Stress."

21. Farquhar, *Knowing Practice*.

22. For ethnographies of medical visualization in American clinical settings, see Saunders, *CT Suite,* and Baim, *Eye to Eye*.

Chapter 2. Things

1. Quoted in dictionary entry on qi in Editing Committee, *Encyclopedic Dictionary*, 58.

2. Heidegger, "The Thing."

3. See Van Fraassen, *Empirical Stance*.

4. And, as Zhang Zai's epigraph reminds us, all these "10,000" things are ever-changing and inter-transforming. See Farquhar and Zhang, *Ten Thousand Things,* for discussions of the *shengsheng huahua* (生生化化 constant genesis and

transformation) of reality as proposed by much classic metaphysics. Given that gods, the dead, sage-kings, bad dreams, and medical patterns of disorder (see below) can be numbered among the 10,000 things, the term "materiality," or *wu*, may be misleading—there is very little left to be "immaterial" and placed in contrast to *wu* concreteness.

5. Latour and Weibel, *Making Things Public.*

6. For example: Bennett, *Vibrant Matter*; Bennett and Connolly, "Crumpled Handkerchief"; Harman, *Prince of Networks*; Ingold, "Re-Thinking the Animate, Re-Animating Thought"; Jullien, *The Propensity of Things*; Bogost, *Alien Phenomenology, or What It's Like to Be a Thing.*

7. This observation is usually attributed to sociologist W. I. Thomas, citing his co-authored book *The Child in America.* Clearly he was influenced by American pragmatists like James and Dewey in making this point.

8. Porkert, *Theoretical Foundations of Chinese Medicine*; Lu and Needham, *Celestial Lancets*; Kaptchuk, *The Web That Has No Weaver*, 35–41; Sivin, *Traditional Medicine in Contemporary China*, 46–53. I particularly value Nathan Sivin's and Ted Kaptchuk's discussions, because they emphasize the activity and multiplicity of qi as both thing and concept.

9. I will follow a somewhat problematic convention in this book by using "TCM" to refer to the modern (post-1955) institutional and epistemological system loosely referred to in China as *zhongyi* 中医 or "Chinese medicine." (The contrasting term in China is *xiyi* 西医, "Western medicine.") This "TCM" is not one thing, nor is it very "traditional," though medicine in China has a long, rich, and hugely diverse history. Modern TCM, moreover, has adopted much from a rather hegemonic bioscience and "Western medicine"—sometimes without noticing the appropriation and adaptation of ideas and objects in translation. Unlike some commentators, who challenge the "authenticity" of TCM as against "classical" medicine in China, in this book I insist on the value of reflecting on the things, thought, and action worlds of TCM, the modern formation to which so many in China are deeply committed.

10. Indeed, in everyday modern standard Chinese, "qi" is a word that refers to air, gas, or breath with no ambiguity or confusion. For a technical treatment, see an influential modern article on the ultimate substantiality of qi, Hong, "Comments on the Hypothesis of Qi."

11. See Huang, "Chang Tsai's Concept of Qi"; Kasoff, *Thought of Chang Tsai.*

12. See Kuriyama, *Expressiveness of the Body*, chapter 6 on the history of winds and qi.

13. Cf. Geaney, *Emergence of Word-Meaning in Early China*.

14. Think about what it would be like to work daily, in the clinic, with a substance that "cannot but" gather *and* scatter according to its own multiple natural propensities. The epigraph from Zhang Zai invites comparison of medical work with *Alice through the Looking Glass*: she must try to play croquet according to an arbitrary queen's rules with a grumpy hedgehog for her ball and a far-from-rigid flamingo for her mallet. Her tools have their own propensities, they are not playing the same game as Alice. As many have emphasized, Chinese doctors must learn to intervene in a world that is in constant transformation.

15. Deng, ed., *Basic Theory of TCM*, 37.

16. Editing Committee, *Encyclopedic Dictionary*, 58.

17. Scorzon, "*Tong* 通 in Clinical Acupuncture Practice," 9.

18. For this point Scorzon cites four clinical research reports from the specialized literature of acupuncture medicine. Qi that can be "gotten" is well-known to practitioners.

19. Scorzon, "*Tong* 通 in Clinical Acupuncture Practice," 11.

20. Some others who have emphasized *tong* or through-passage in discussion of Chinese medicine are Scheid and Virag, "Introduction to History of Science," and Zhang, *Transforming Emotions with Chinese Medicine*.

21. Scorzon, "*Tong* 通 in Clinical Acupuncture Practice," 4.

22. Ibid., 5.

23. Ibid.

24. Fleck, *Genesis and Development of a Scientific Fact*. See also Barbara Herrnstein Smith's sustained engagement with Fleck's historical vision: *Practicing Relativism in the Anthropocene*.

25. *Treponema pallidum p.* is, according to Wikipedia, a pretty inadequate creature, a parasite on human hosts, and very short-lived and slow growing due to its small genome. See Wikipedia, s.v. "Syphilis," last modified January 15, 2019, 16:03, https://en.wikipedia.org/wiki/Syphilis.

26. Lei, *Neither Donkey nor Horse*. Making a distinction between theory and practice in medicine is a modern concern, though Chinese historians of medicine tend to use it as a timeless principle through which they can sort the ancient canon and the whole literature of drugs, cases, and ancillary fields like climatology and cosmology. Thus modern scholars think of the *Inner Canon of the Yellow Emperor* (*Huangdi Neijing* 黄帝内经) as the "theoretical classic" and consider the *Treatise on Cold Disorders* (*Shanghan Lun* 伤寒论) to be the "clinical classic."

27. Much has been written in English about dynamic and non-unitary forms of embodiment that become visible through Chinese medicine. See, for example, Farquhar, "Multiplicity, Point of View, and Responsibility"; Hsu, "Biological in the Cultural"; Schipper, *Taoist Body;* Kaptchuk, *Web That Has No Weaver.*

28. Some scholars have shown that various kinds of traditional medicine were legally recognized by the Indian state in the early part of the twentieth century, and India thus presents an interesting case of long-standing Asian medical pluralism (Leslie, "Ambiguities of Medical Revivalism"). But only China offers an early instance of state support for the extensive institutionalization of a non-Western medical system. See Lampton, *Politics of Medicine in China,* and Taylor, *Chinese Medicine in Early Communist China,* for some explanations about why this interesting historical turn was politically necessary.

29. Some of them specialized in salvaging and sorting out the classical "basic theory" of traditional Chinese medicine. One of the fascinating developments arising from this mid-century development of Chinese medicine was, thus, a great deal of very thoughtful philosophizing. The "theory" of TCM, restored to national dignity especially in the 1980s, was broken out and (re)written by curriculum designers, textbook committees, health services policy makers, historians, and—most of all, I believe—senior clinical practitioners. See Farquhar, "Rewriting Traditional Medicine."

30. See Farquhar, "Metaphysics at the Bedside" and "Knowledge in Translation."

31. I am indebted to Barry Saunders for this gloss of diagnosis and for many interesting discussions of his attention to "cutting" as both a material and a logical aspect of biomedical knowledge.

32. But many, also, do not center *bianzheng lunzhi* in this way. The formation was then, and is now, official but not entirely hegemonic.

33. Both Scheid, *Currents of Tradition,* and Karchmer, "Slow Medicine," have shown in historical research that *bianzheng lunzhi* is a relatively recent model of TCM clinical knowing. My description here is quite deliberately full of ideologically colored recent keywords—in translation—used by the teachers and senior clinicians active in Chinese TCM settings. Examples are experience, practice, and style of thought. On representing and intervening, see Ian Hacking's discussion of scientific method by that name.

34. Ou, ed., *Chinese-English Dictionary of Traditional Chinese Medicine,* s.v. 证候, 258. This is my translation from the Chinese side of the page in this bilingual source. The English translation provided in the dictionary is a bit murkier.

35. One dominant synthesis was to argue that every pattern is a name for a stage of development within the nosological/ontological space occupied by one biomedical disease.

36. James, *Pragmatism*, 252.

37. Deng, ed., *Practical TCM Diagnosis*.

38. See Jensen, "New Ontologies?" for a discussion of some theoretical commitments to the object "withdrawn" from knowledge of it. Also see Daston and Galison, *Objectivity*, on the paired historical emergence of both objects and subjects.

39. I like it that *duixiang* is ungendered in popular vernacular; it is hard to gloss in English since one has to use the awkward phrase "girlfriend or boyfriend," or the ambiguous "partner," to translate it more or less correctly. "The image we face" is no less awkward, of course. But the notion of the thing, understood through Heidegger, "The Thing," and Latour and Weibel, *Making Things Public*, actually corresponds quite nicely.

40. See Bowker and Star, *Sorting Things Out*, on the International Classification of Diseases.

41. See Farquhar, "Objects, Processes, and Female Infertility." Colin Garon has written a highly relevant study of "concrescences" in Chinese medical clinics, drawing on the writing of Lu Guangxin and observing an increasing reliance on anatomical imaging in TCM clinics in Beijing. See Garon, "Clinical Concrescences."

42. See Hamdy, *Our Bodies Belong to God.*

43. Arguably, gross anatomy is also increasingly a bore in biomedical training, except perhaps for aspiring surgeons. Human dissection labs are—some say—slowly being phased out in favor of using digitized virtual male and female bodies for online training, and anatomy is no longer an active research field in its own right.

44. Farquhar, "Objects, Processes, and Female Infertility."

45. They even refer to brains, though the functions of brains in the Chinese medical body are more than a little hard to sort out from the medical archive. See Farquhar, "Chinese Medicine and the Life of the Mind."

46. Somewhere along the line I acquired, in a toy store, small pink plastic renditions of some internal organs: a heart, doubled kidneys and lungs, a stomach with some gastric tubing. Puzzling over them at the beginning, it took me a while to figure out which was which, and they still confuse my guests who come to my house to play. Organs are far from self-evident objects, which is why dissectors need guidebooks to tell them what they are seeing in the cadaver.

47. Sivin, *Traditional Medicine in Modern China.*

48. Farquhar, *Knowing Practice*, 73.

49. Translations of body parts in this section of the chapter are drawn from Wiseman and Feng, *Practical Dictionary of Chinese Medicine*.

50. See Ames, *Art of Rulership*. This important study incorporates a translation of Book Nine of the *Huainanzi*, a crucial "Daoist" work of the second century BCE. Book Nine is entitled *zhushu* 主术, literally the arts of ruling. Also see Zhang Dong, "Preface" (translated in appendix 2).

51. This is the question asked by Shigehisa Kuriyama in his brilliant comparative study of ancient Chinese and classical Greek medicine: *The Expressiveness of the Body*.

52. Thomas and Thomas, *Child in America*, 571–72.

53. Here I refer to Heidegger's distinction in "The Thing" between "objects" ready-to-hand (but out of our awareness) and "things" that are present-at-hand, salient for us. Also see Bruno Latour's opening discussion in *Pandora's Hope* of the challenged but nevertheless irrefutable reality of a world that is "socially constructed." And "propensities" is François Jullien's translation for *shi* 势, a notion as important in medicine (which Jullien ignores) as in the aesthetic philosophy he mainly reads. Law and Lin, "Provincializing STS," have discussed the importance of propensity in TCM.

Chapter 3. Thought

1. Liao, *Medicine Is Thought*. This author, Liao Yuqun, found the statement "Medicine is thought" in *The Book of the Later Han*, a fifth-century history, and re-entered it into discussion in Chinese medicine circles in the 2000s. The phrase is now often repeated in contemporary commentaries on the value of Chinese medicine beyond the conventionally recognized efficacies of its drugs and needles.

2. James, *Essays in Radical Empiricism;* Kohn, *How Forests Think*; Montgomery, *Soul of an Octopus*.

3. There was widespread excitement throughout China when Dr. Tu Youyou won the 2015 Nobel Prize in medicine for her Chinese group's development of an anti-malarial drug, the herbal basis of which was "discovered" in the Chinese medical archive. Bioscientific facts constructed in China are rare indeed and always worthy of comment among nationalists!

4. As argued in chapter 2, *bianzheng lunzhi* can be seen as a schooled approach to gathering the pattern of disorder into (temporary and contingent) existence. On

gathering, see Heidegger, "The Thing," and Zhuang, *Zhuangzi*, 380. This chapter will concentrate on the knowing rather than the acting side of figure 1, and chapter 4 will return to the whole process as seen through the lens of action.

5. See Smith, *Discerning the Subject*, on the particular implications of the verb I am privileging here, "discerning."

6. See Kaptchuk, *Web That Has No Weaver*, 59–60. Yi 意, here translated as "thought," is not just cognition but intention, awareness of potentials, a perceptive stance that leans toward things and events, a gathering attentiveness, and more.

7. This radical understanding of "thought" is reminiscent of the pragmatist problematization of the commonsense distinction between "thought" and "thing." For those who would insist that medicine is also a lot of things (drugs, microscopes, viruses, diseases, etc.), a practice philosophy asks that the distance between thinking ideas and perceiving things be narrowed. See James, *Essays in Radical Empiricism*, especially chapters 1–3.

8. Xie Guan is better known in the field as the first and most accomplished editor of the *Encyclopedic Dictionary of Chinese Medicine*, a multivolume authoritative encyclopedia of Chinese medicine, which is still being produced. His 1935 history, *Sources and Currents of Chinese Medicine*, was loaded with historical information and wise interpretation. Above all, it was a defense of a plural tradition in the face of destructive modernization and scientization efforts to standardize and reductively explain. Perhaps the book's politically situated historical character partly accounts for its contemporary obscurity. For a more recent and popular alternative, see Ren, *On China's Medical History*.

9. Lei, *Neither Donkey nor Horse*.

10. These considerations are reflected in the translations and commentaries in several editions of *A Source Book in Chinese Philosophy*, where it is not only Zhu Xi's treatment of *li* that is under consideration. But in this authoritative teaching resource, *li* tends to be translated throughout as "principle," no doubt for consistency. See both the Chan and the De Bary and Bloom editions of the *Source Book*.

11. See Dictionary Editing Group, *Contemporary Chinese Dictionary* (1978), s.v. "*li* 理." Interestingly, the specialized TCM dictionaries do not define the single morpheme *li* 理 at all. Rather, the word is treated by those sources, by omission, as a commonsense word in everyday Chinese.

12. Drug formulas are composed in very structured ways, with the properties and quantities of each component carefully balanced, usually by weight in grams, within

the written prescription. The most common verb for designing an herbal medicine prescription is *chufang* 处方, which refers to positioning drugs relative to each other in a compound formula.

13. But see Lei, *Neither Donkey nor Horse.*

14. Liao Yuqun argues, in his *Medicine Is Thought*, that the word we are translating as thought, for the ancient writers most often referred to perceptiveness (*zhuyili* 注意力). See Geaney, *On the Epistemology of the Senses*, for a highly relevant study of perceptiveness in early Chinese philosophy.

15. James, *Essays in Radical Empiricism*, 34.

16. Dr. Ping lectured on this point to our group, and it's in the textbooks; but it is unlikely that any one physician actually uses all of these possibilities in his or her practice. There is considerable variation in the sets of qualities and sites usually examined by different doctors.

17. William James in "A World of Pure Experience" discusses the only superficial differences between "direct" and "indirect" experience; his "radical empiricism" is akin to the insistence of Chinese medical people that they "take experience to be the main thing" (Farquhar, *Knowing Practice*). Indeed, the word for empiricism in Chinese is "experience-ism," *jingyanzhuyi* 经验主义. Possibly this term originated with John Dewey's teaching in China.

18. I write these lines in late August, in an unusually hot and humid Chicago. Those of us whose most chronic TCM complaint is "spleen deficiency" understand the seasonal timing of rheumatic symptoms (*fengshi bing* 风湿病) associated with the spleen visceral system (which, by the way, "hates damp"). Our systemic symptoms are much worse in the damp, heat-afflicted season of late summer (*shu* 暑). However skeptical one might have been when first diagnosed, after a few years of suffering so predictably, one is increasingly persuaded of the correctness of this TCM pattern.

19. Qin, *Introduction to Chinese Medicine*. The edition I have is a tenth printing of 635,000-plus copies, made in 1983. The book is still in wide circulation after many more printings. See Scheid, *Currents of Tradition*, for Qin Bowei's historical importance.

20. I include this sentence mainly to remind any habitual readers of modern Chinese discourses that this is indeed a 1959 source.

21. Qin Bowei in this "introduction" to the field defines, refines, and explains the methodology of discerning patterns and determining therapies (*bianzheng lunzhi*) at a crucial moment in the development of this model as a ruling logic for the field,

all the while linking this clinical methodology to *li fa fang yao* and insisting on certain Chinese specificities of reasoning and knowing. My approach here is similar to his; compare figure 1 and box 2 for the analogous approach.

22. See Zhang Dong's critique of the gap between self and thing (*wuwo fenli* 物我分离) that he sees as presumed by a Western dualist epistemology, in appendix 2.

23. Liao, *Medicine Is Thought*, 42.

24. "Sources" is a more powerful notion than "cause" for understanding physiology and pathology, as I hope will be clear in this section. Also see appendix 1.

25. Farquhar and Zhang, *Ten Thousand Things*, chapter 4. I invoke "nature" here in awareness that the Chinese term in use among Chinese doctors is *da ziran* (大自然), the great spontaneity.

26. Zhuang, *Zhuangzi*, chapter 18.

27. Zhang, *Original Qi, Vital Machine*, ii.

28. Ibid., vii.

29. Ibid., viii.

30. If we were to consult a standard "TCM Theory" textbook about "original qi," we would be likely to find that it originates in the "former heaven," or innate endowment, of the kidney visceral system and that its allied organ is the "gate of life" (*mingmen* 命门). And original qi thrives when it is fed by the essential nutrients transformed by the "latter heaven" of the spleen-stomach system and the triple burner system (*sanjiao* 三焦). See Yin, *Basic Theory of Chinese Medicine*, 57.

31. Lau and Ames, trans., *Yuan Dao*. Lau and Ames here translate and comment on the preface of the *Huainanzi* (second century BCE), revealing the logic of thinking cosmogonically for that same "axial age" that interests Zhang Dong. Lau and Ames are able to draw out the many implications of "the three gives birth to the myriads," which neither Zhang Dong in his preface nor I in this chapter have space to do.

32. Mao, "On Practice," in *Selected Works*.

33. Here I omit several other important analytics, notably the "Six Warps" analysis preferred by doctors of the Cold Damage current. But there are others.

34. Though there are blood depletion patterns, qi depletion is much more common. Because of the intimate qi/blood relationship in which qi drives blood and blood supports qi, signs expressing a failure of blood functions (especially heart visceral system functions) almost by definition are rooted in a more determining shortfall of qi activity.

35. Deng, ed., *Practical TCM Diagnosis*, 215.

36. The modern Chinese words for physiology (*shenglixue* 生理学) and pathology (*binglixue* 病理学) incorporate that pattern-word, *li,* discussed above and in box 2. The literal translation would be "study of the patterns of life" and "study of the patterns of illness."

37. Liao, *Medicine Is Thought*, 46.

38. Ibid., 47.

Chapter 4. Action

1. Latour, *Pasteurization of France*.

2. Latour and Woolgar, *Laboratory Life*; Latour, *Pandora's Hope*.

3. Fleck, *Genesis and Development*.

4. Croizier, *Traditional Medicine in Modern China*; Lei, *Neither Donkey nor Horse*; Lampton, *Politics of Medicine in China*; Taylor, *Chinese Medicine in Early Communist China*; Karchmer, "Slow Medicine."

5. These were the early years of the "Chinese [Reform Era] Dream," which continues to be more assumed than articulated. See Farquhar, "You Had to Have Been There."

6. See Smith, *Contingencies of Value*, for an extended analysis of the epistemological and ethical relativities of practical science. She critiques the objectivist axiologies that would posit universal criteria of value and embraces a certain relativism in a way that I found immensely useful, as I was writing *Knowing Practice*, trying to come to terms with the profound pragmatism of TCM.

7. Mao, *Serve the People*; Sidel and Sidel, *Serve the People*.

8. Descriptive observations like these tend to invite comparison with the life and practice of biomedical clinics. In my view, much of what happens between doctor and patient in TCM is quite similar to practice in biomedicine, partly because a number of institutional forms (such as the form of the case record and the taking of a "history") were borrowed by TCM modernizers half a century ago from standard practices in the United States and Europe. Further, Canguilhem in *The Normal and the Pathological* emphasized the social (rather than scientific) specificities that determined the telos of medical work, even the identification of the pathological, in mid-twentieth-century European clinics. But it remains important here that, in the TCM clinic, the patient's own understanding of what is wrong is so closely attended to. Chinese doctors seldom suspect their patients of being hypochondriacs

or malingerers. To understand the "problem" of the judgment of hypochondria in biomedical clinics would require field research, and I hesitate to speculate on differences noticed only through experience as a very particular patient.

9. See Hacking, *Representing and Intervening*, on the rather ideological separation in the philosophy of science of these two kinds of action.

10. See Farquhar, "Time and Text," for a discussion of the ongoing tinkering and tweaking typical of TCM clinical action. On birthing and transforming, see chapter 3. Also see chapter 4 in Farquhar and Zhang, *Ten Thousand Things*.

11. Shifts in China's public health financing, institutional hierarchies, and regulatory environment since the 1990s have encouraged the founding of many private clinics and hospitals in the cities where TCM expertise tends to be concentrated. Because patients pay a larger percentage of the cost of services offered in these private facilities, considerable effort is expended by management to attract patients and make them feel they are receiving all the benefits of the practice and experience of senior doctors in TCM. In such clinics, computers keep patient records and control pharmacy inventory and drug dispensing, and laboratory kitchens prepare microwavable medicinal decoctions for the convenience of busy clients. But there is little other "high technology" on offer, and the aesthetic of a simple consultation space and a scholarly tradition is self-consciously maintained. Zhang Dong in his preface (appendix 2) speaks of the "plain and simple" character of the most classic medicine. His point is in keeping with popular ways of appreciating the special character of TCM.

12. Liao, *Medicine Is Thought*, 47.

13. See Feuchtwang, *Anthropology of Religion*, as well as other works by Feuchtwang for discussion of "ling efficacy." Also see Farquhar, *Knowing Practice*, on the *ling* or *linghuo* 灵活 flexibility of the skilled Chinese doctor. Elsewhere in his book *Medicine Is Thought*, Liao Yuqun also makes much of *linghuo* adeptness on the part of TCM doctors.

14. Suzanne Cochrane in a personal communication has reminded me, from the perspective of an anglophone Chinese medical practitioner, that this word *tiao* (调) is often better translated as "attune." The attuning of whole bodies and lives in the practice of TCM is arguably a more ambitious undertaking than the adjusting referred to in this tenth-century text. The latter source refers to something "from outside" performing an adjustment to an illness, which is perhaps a more partial process than the holistic body that can be "attuned."

15. Nappi, *Monkey and the Inkpot*. Nappi shows that Li Shizhen inhabited the very limit of thought in use, with his "minute participation" in metamorphosis and its patterns.

16. Andrew Pickering, in *Constructing Quarks* and *The Mangle of Practice*, has innovated in science studies with his detailed readings of knowledge in practice, which are very relevant to this book. See also Scheid, *Chinese Medicine in Contemporary China*, whose treatment of "plurality and synthesis" in Chinese medicine invokes Pickering's approach to emergence in scientific practice.

17. A reminder: I use the analytic method of the eight rubrics here only to make the patterning and pathology-countering logic of Chinese medicine thought clear. Practicing doctors are unlikely to rely on this simplistic method alone.

18. I noted above that yinyang and the five phases are widely taken to be the most central "theoretical foundations" of Chinese medicine. Critics abound, however, arguing that five phases classifications and dynamics, as described here, are pure superstition and cannot be part of a scientific modern medicine. Even some theoretically inclined practitioners of classical Chinese medicine have been known to pooh-pooh the logic of the five phases, arguing that any such classification system is wooden and unresponsive to the specificities of illness in the clinic. Senior leader of the field Deng Tietao, however, has defended this "system," arguing that he finds the production and restraint relations between the phases very useful for thinking about the dynamics of the ruling visceral systems in bodies. Deng, "Dialectical Factors" and "Reconsidering Dialectical Factors."

19. *Juan* 2 of the "Plain Questions" (part one of the *Yellow Emperor's Inner Canon, Huangdi Neijing* 黄帝内经), cited in Farquhar, *Knowing Practice*, 31.

20. Both Renée Fox, *Experiment Perilous*, and Katherine Montgomery, *How Doctors Think*, have written brilliantly about chronic uncertainty in biomedical practice. In biomedical clinics, treatment protocols (see Berg, *Rationalizing Medical Work*) and disease classifications (see Bowker and Star, *Sorting Things Out*, and Bowker, *Memory Practices in the Sciences*) are expected to reduce doubt and improve accountability in diagnosis and therapeutics. Modern Chinese medicine also uses such tools, but many seasoned clinicians distrust and resent them.

21. Farquhar, "Time and Text"; Furth et al., eds., *Thinking with Cases*.

22. Chinese medical people, when they compare TCM to biomedicine, often scoff at a certain literal-mindedness they take to be characteristic of biomedicine. They say: "Western medicine doctors are too direct. When the head hurts they treat

the head, when the foot hurts they treat the foot. TCM is much more subtle, it seeks the deep and non-proximal roots of disorder."

23. See appendix 1 on the question of causation in medicine. Here Deng's mention of the "reasons" for disease and the "illness essence," as well as his attention to "cause," make clear reference to ontological disease and its causes, even though he is primarily urging a different approach, the discernment of a pattern and the seeking of root sources in an ongoing pattern of emergence.

24. Deng, ed., *Basic Theory of TCM*, 155.

25. Ibid.

26. See Heidegger, "The Thing," on the subject of the thing that is present at hand.

27. Strictly speaking, the question was first posed by N. G. Chernyshevsky as the title of an 1880s novel and then used again as a title by Leo Tolstoy for his essays. But it is Lenin's polemic, *What Is to Be Done? Burning Questions of Our Time,* that was most noticed in China.

28. Murthy, *Political Philosophy of Zhang Taiyan.*

29. Lu, *The Way,* 5.

30. Of course the word I translate as "thing" here is *duixiang* 对象.

31. Lu, *The Way,* 7.

32. Mao, "On Practice."

33. Lu, *The Way,* 5.

Appendix 1: Comparison and Causation

1. Patricia Kaufert and John O'Neil, "Analysis of a Dialogue on Risks in Childbirth."

2. As Ted Kaptchuk points out, this everyday wisdom for moderns with access to biomedical care stems from the relatively recent development of infectious disease management with antibacterials, the classic magic bullet of modern medical history (*Web That Has No Weaver,* 47–48, 196). See also Allan M. Brandt, *No Magic Bullet.*

3. Kaptchuk, *Web That Has No Weaver,* 115–37, relates his discussion of the problem of causation to this down-to-earth question, although he sometimes phrases it in his preferred TCM terms: "Why is there disharmony?" See also page 118.

4. E. E. Evans-Pritchard, *Witchcraft, Oracles and Magic among the Azande.*

5. Lloyd and Sivin, *Way and the Word,* 160.

6. Young, "Discourse on Stress."

7. Kaptchuk, *Web That Has No Weaver,* 261.

8. Ibid., 13.

9. Sivin, *Traditional Medicine in Contemporary China,* 274n2.

10. In philosophy of science there is, of course, a great deal of writing about causation (and determinism, and freedom from determination), much of it noting the arbitrariness, in applied sciences like medicine, of assigning the role of cause to only one of many simultaneously active factors or agents. Here I confine my attention to China studies comparativists, some of whom have examined the problem of cause, and "the Chinese" disinterest in it, in considerable detail. One interesting discussion to which I cannot do justice here is quite classic: see Needham, *Science and Civilization in China,* vol. 2, 280 et passim, where he provides a fascinating reading of the metaphysics of Dong Zhongshu (Tung Chung-Shu in his romanization, 179–104 BCE). In place of the "external causation" or "subordinative thinking characteristic of European science," Needham and the authorities he cites speak of "inductance" or "a kind of mysterious resonance." Interactive resonance as causation in systems of affinity and contrast among "the myriad things" is an attractive idea when we think about Chinese medicine. But the Han Confucian Dong Zhongshu aside, resonance (*ganying* 感应) is far from being the only approach to causation and efficacy found in the philosophical literature. François Jullien's work on efficacy (*A Treatise on Efficacy*) and propensity (*The Propensity of Things*) is highly relevant here.

11. In my first long period of following clinical work in a hospital of Chinese medicine, I took to asking doctors, "What was the cause of this illness we are currently treating?" Several times my teachers' expression of frustration with my question went as follows: "Cause? How would I know? Ask the patient, they might have an idea." We were, of course, using the term *bingyin* to talk about cause, and it is interesting to me that they thought of this "illness factor" as temporally displaced, i.e., having been in play as an origin point or cause at an earlier time and thus no longer relevant to pathology and physiology.

12. Sivin, *Traditional Medicine in Contemporary China,* 274n2.

13. Kaptchuk makes this point as well, *Web That Has No Weaver,* 116.

14. Beijing Zhongyi Xueyuan, chief ed., *Fundamentals of Chinese Medicine,* 52. Quotations in the following paragraphs are also from this page.

15. Mao, "On Contradiction," is the chief source of this logic for 1980s Chinese medicine.

16. See, for example, Kaptchuk, *Web That Has No Weaver,* and Zhang, *Philosophical Foundations of Chinese Medicine.*

17. François Jullien has recast "efficacity" at length in several stimulating studies, but he has seldom drawn on Chinese medical materials. See especially *The Propensity of Things* and *A Treatise on Efficacy.*

Appendix 2: Yes, Medicine Is Thought!

1. Zhang Dong, 张东. 元气 神机：先秦中医之道 *Yuanqi Shenji: Xianqin Zhongyi zhi Dao* [Original Qi, Vital Machine] (Xi'an: World Book Publishers, 2016).

2. This translation follows, loosely, that provided by Michael Stanley-Baker in "Health and Philosophy in Pre- and Early Imperial China." I thank him for sending me this forthcoming paper at exactly the moment I needed it. My translation attempts to highlight Zhang Dong's interest in the inscription, so it differs a little from Dr. Stanley-Baker's.

Bibliography

Ames, Roger T. *The Art of Rulership: A Study of Ancient Chinese Political Thought.* Albany: State University of New York Press, 1994.

Anderson, Warwick, and Ian R. Mackay. *Intolerant Bodies: A Short History of Autoimmunity.* Baltimore, MD: Johns Hopkins University Press, 2014.

Asad, Talal. 1986. "The Concept of Cultural Translation in British Social Anthropology." In *Writing Culture: The Poetics and Politics of Ethnography,* edited by James Clifford and George E. Marcus, 141–64. Berkeley: University of California Press, 1986.

Baim, Adam. "Eye to Eye: Visuality and the Work of Vision in Ophthalmology." PhD diss., University of Chicago, 2018.

Bakhtin, M. M. "Discourse in the Novel." In *The Dialogic Imagination: Four Essays,* edited by Michael Holquist, translated by Caryl Emerson and Michael Holquist, 269–422. Austin: University of Texas Press, 1981.

Beijing Zhongyi Xueyuan 北京中医学院, chief ed., 中医学基础 *Zhongyixue Jichu* [Fundamentals of Chinese Medicine]. Shanghai: Shanghai Science and Technology Press, 1978.

Bennett, Jane. *Vibrant Matter: A Political Ecology of Things.* Durham, NC: Duke University Press, 2010.

Bennett, Jane, and William Connolly. "The Crumpled Handkerchief." In *Time and History in Deleuze and Serre,* edited by Bernd Herzogenrath, 153–71. London: Continuum, 2012.

Berg, Marc. *Rationalizing Medical Work: Decision-Support Techniques and Medical Practices.* Cambridge, MA: MIT Press, 1997.

Bogost, Ian. *Alien Phenomenology, or What It's Like to Be a Thing*. Minneapolis: University of Minnesota Press, 2012.

Bowker, Geoffrey C. *Memory Practices in the Sciences*. Cambridge, MA: MIT Press, 2005.

Bowker, Geoffrey C., and Susan Leigh Star. *Sorting Things Out: Classification and Its Consequences*. Cambridge, MA: MIT Press, 1999.

Brandt, Allan M. *No Magic Bullet: A Social History of Venereal Disease in the United States since 1880*. New York: Oxford University Press, 1985.

Canguilhem, Georges. *The Normal and the Pathological*. Translated by Carolyn R. Fawcett in collaboration with Robert S. Cohen. New York: Zone Books, 1989.

Chan, Wing-Tsit, trans. *A Source Book in Chinese Philosophy*. Princeton, NJ: Princeton University Press, 1963.

Connolly, William E. *Pluralism*. Durham, NC: Duke University Press, 2005.

Croizier, Ralph C. *Traditional Medicine in Modern China: Science, Nationalism, and the Tensions of Cultural Change*. Cambridge, MA: Harvard University Press, 1968.

Daston, Lorraine. "Introduction: The Coming into Being of Scientific Objects." In *Biographies of Scientific Objects*, edited by Lorraine Daston, 1–14. Chicago: University of Chicago Press, 2000.

Daston, Lorraine, and Peter Galison. *Objectivity*. New York: Zone Books, 2007.

De Bary, William Theodore, and Irene Bloom, eds. *Sources of Chinese Tradition: From Earliest Times to 1600*, 2nd ed. New York: Columbia University Press, 1999.

Deng, Tietao 邓铁涛, ed. 中医基础理论 *Zhongyi Jichu Lilun* [Basic Theory of TCM]. Guangzhou: Guangdong Science and Technology Press, 1982.

———. "中医五行学说的辩证法因素 *Zhongyi Wuxing Xueshuo de Bianzhengfa Yinsu* [Dialectical Factors in Five Phases Thought]." In 学说探讨与临证 *Xueshuo Tantao yu Linzheng* [Clinical and Scholarly Exploration], 4–7. Guangzhou: Guangdong Science and Technology Press, 1981.

———, ed. 使用中医诊断学 *Shiyong Zhongyi Zhenduanxue* [Practical TCM Diagnosis]. Shanghai: Shanghai Science and Technology Press, 1983.

———. "再论中医五行学说的辩证法因素 *Zailun Zhongyi Wuxing Xue-shuo de Bianzhengfa Yinsu* [Reconsidering Dialectical Factors in Five Phases Thought]. In 学说探讨与临证 *Xueshuo Tantao yu Linzheng* [Clinical and Scholarly Explorations], 8–15. Guangzhou: Guangdong Science and Technology Press, 1981.

Dictionary Editing Group, Chinese Academy of Social Sciences Language Institute, ed. 现代汉语词典 *Xiandai Hanyu Cidian* [Contemporary Chinese Dictionary]. Beijing: Commercial Press, 1978.

Doniger, Wendy. *Against Dharma: Dissent in the Ancient Indian Sciences of Sex and Politics*. New Haven, CT: Yale University Press, 2018.

Douglas, Mary. *Thinking in Circles: An Essay on Ring Composition*. New Haven, CT: Yale University Press, 2007.

Durkheim, Émile. *The Elementary Forms of the Religious Life*. Translated by Karen E. Fields. New York: Free Press, 1995.

Editing Committee of Encyclopedic Dictionary of Chinese Medicine 中医大辞典编辑委, ed. 中医大辞典 基础理论分册 *Zhongyi Daci-dian Jichu Lilun Fence* [Encyclopedic Dictionary of Chinese Medicine: Basic Theory]. Beijing: People's Health Press, 1982.

Evans-Pritchard, E. E. *Witchcraft, Oracles, and Magic among the Azande*. Oxford: Clarendon Press, 1937.

Farquhar, Judith. "Chinese Medicine and the Life of the Mind: Are Brains Necessary?" *North Carolina Medical Journal* 59, no. 3 (May–June 1998): 188–90.

———. *Knowing Practice: The Clinical Encounter of Chinese Medicine*. Boulder, CO: Westview Press, 1994.

———. "Knowledge in Translation: Global Science, Local Things." In *Medicine and the Politics of Knowledge*, edited by Susan Levine, 153–70. Cape Town, South Africa: HSRC Press, 2012.

———. "Metaphysics at the Bedside." In *Historical Epistemology and the Making of Modern Chinese Medicine*, edited by Howard Chiang, 219–36. Manchester: Manchester University Press, 2015.

———. "Multiplicity, Point of View, and Responsibility in Traditional Chinese Medicine." In *Body, Subjectivity and Power in China*, edited by Angela Zito and Tani E. Barlow, 78–99. Chicago: University of Chicago Press, 1994.

———. "Objects, Processes, and Female Infertility in Chinese Medicine." *Medical Anthropology Quarterly* 5, no. 4 (December 1991): 370–99.

———. "Rewriting Traditional Medicine in Post-Maoist China." In *Knowledge and the Scholarly Medical Traditions*, edited by Don Bates, 251–76. Cambridge: Cambridge University Press, 1995.

———. "Time and Text: Approaching Contemporary Chinese Medicine through Analysis of a Case." In *Paths to Asian Medical Knowledge*, edited by Charles Leslie and Allan Young, 62–73. Berkeley: University of California Press, 1992.

———. "You Had to Have Been There: Laughing at Lunch about the Chinese Dream." *Critical Inquiry* 43, no. 2 (Winter 2017): 451–65.

Farquhar, Judith, and Qicheng Zhang. *Ten Thousand Things: Nurturing Life in Contemporary Beijing*. New York: Zone Books, 2012.

Feuchtwang, Stephan. *The Anthropology of Religion, Charisma, and Ghosts: Chinese Lessons for Adequate Theory*. Berlin: W. de Gruyter, 2010.

Fleck, Ludwik. *Genesis and Development of a Scientific Fact*. Chicago: University of Chicago Press, 1979.

Foucault, Michael. Introduction to *The Normal and the Pathological*, by Georges Canguilhem, 7–24. Translated by Carolyn R. Fawcett in collaboration with Robert S. Cohen. New York: Zone Books, 1989.

———. *The Order of Things: An Archaeology of the Human Sciences*. New York: Vintage Books, 1994.

Fox, Renée C. *Experiment Perilous: Physicians and Patients Facing the Unknown*. Glencoe, IL: Free Press, 1959.

Furth, Charlotte, Judith T. Zeitlin, and Ping-chen Hsiung, eds. *Thinking with Cases: Specialist Knowledge in Chinese Cultural History*. Honolulu: University of Hawai'i Press, 2007.

Garon, Colin. "Clinical Concrescences: Integration in Contemporary Chinese Medicine Gynecology." BA thesis, History and Philosophy of Science Program, University of Chicago, 2018.

Geaney, Jane. *The Emergence of Word-Meaning in Early China: A Normative Model for Words.* Albany: State University of New York Press, forthcoming.

———. *On the Epistemology of the Senses in Early Chinese Thought.* Honolulu: University of Hawai'i Press, 2002.

Geertz, Clifford. *Islam Observed: Religious Development in Morocco and Indonesia.* New Haven, CT: Yale University Press, 1968.

Hacking, Ian. *Representing and Intervening: Introductory Topics in the Philosophy of Natural Science.* Cambridge: Cambridge University Press, 1983.

Hamdy, Sherine. *Our Bodies Belong to God: Organ Transplants, Islam, and the Struggle for Human Dignity in Egypt.* Berkeley: University of California Press, 2012.

Harman, Graham. *Prince of Networks: Bruno Latour and Metaphysics.* Prahran, Australia: Re.press, 2009.

Hart, Roger. "On the Problem of Chinese Science." In *The Science Studies Reader*, edited by Mario Biagioli, 123–30. New York: Routledge, 1999.

Heidegger, Martin. "The Thing." In *Poetry, Language, Thought*, translated by Albert Hofstadter, 161–84. New York: Harper & Row, 1971.

Hong, Menghu 洪梦浒. 评"气"基表物质又表机能的两义说 *Ping qi ji biao wuzhi you biao jineng de liangyi shuo* [Comments on the Hypothesis of "Vital Energy (Qi)" Denoting Both Material and Function]. 中医杂志 *Zhongyi zazhi* 24, no. 3 (1983): 4–7.

Hsu, Elisabeth. "The Biological in the Cultural: The Five Agents and the Body Ecologic in Chinese Medicine." In *Holistic Anthropology: Emergence and Convergence*, edited by David Parkin and Stanley Ulijaszek, 91–126. New York: Berghann Books, 2007.

Huang, Siu-chi. "Chang Tsai's Concept of Qi." *Philosophy East and West* 18, no. 4 (1968): 247–60.

Ingold, Tim. "Re-Thinking the Animate, Re-Animating Thought." *Ethnos* 71, no. 1 (2006): 9–20.

James, William. *Essays in Radical Empiricism.* New York: Longmans, Green, 1912. Republished by Mineola, NY: Dover Publications, 2003. Page references are to the 2003 edition.

———. *A Pluralistic Universe: Hibbert Lectures at Manchester College on the Present Situation in Philosophy.* New York: Longmans, Green, 1909.

———. *Pragmatism, a New Name for Some Old Ways of Thinking: Popular Lectures on Philosophy.* New York: Longmans, Green, 1907.

———. "A World of Pure Experience." In *Essays in Radical Empiricism,* 21–47. New York: Longmans, Green, 1912. Republished by Mineola, NY: Dover Publications, 2003. Page references are to the 2003 edition.

Jensen, Casper Bruun. "New Ontologies? Reflections on Some Recent 'Turns' in STS, Anthropology and Philosophy." *Social Anthropology* 25, no. 4 (2017): 525–45.

Jullien, François. *The Propensity of Things: Toward a History of Efficacy in China,* translated by Janet Lloyd. New York: Zone Books, 1995.

———. *A Treatise on Efficacy: Between Western and Chinese Thinking.* Honolulu: University of Hawai'i Press, 2004.

Kaptchuk, Ted J. *The Web That Has No Weaver: Understanding Chinese Medicine.* Lincolnwood, IL: Contemporary Books, 2000.

Karchmer, Eric. "Slow Medicine: How Chinese Medicine Became Efficacious Only for Chronic Conditions." In *Worlds of Chinese Medicine: Historical Epistemology and Transnational Cultural Politics,* edited by Howard Hsueh. Forthcoming.

Kasoff, Ira E. *The Thought of Chang Tsai, 1020–1077.* Cambridge: Cambridge University Press, 1984.

Kaufert, Patricia, and John O'Neil. "Analysis of a Dialogue on Risks in Childbirth: Clinicians, Epidemiologists, and Inuit Women." In *Knowledge, Power, and Practice: The Anthropology of Medicine and Everyday Life,* edited by Shirley Lindenbaum and Margaret Lock, 32–54. Berkeley: University of California Press, 1993.

Kohn, Eduardo. *How Forests Think: Toward an Anthropology beyond the Human.* Berkeley: University of California Press, 2013.

Kuriyama, Shigehisa. *The Expressiveness of the Body and the Divergence of Greek and Chinese Medicine.* New York: Zone Books, 1999.

Lampton, David M. *The Politics of Medicine in China: The Policy Process, 1949–1977.* Boulder, CO: Westview Press, 1977.

Landecker, Hannah. "Metabolism, Autonomy, Individuality." In *Biological Individuality: Integrating Scientific, Philosophical, and Historical Perspectives*, edited by Scott Lidgard and Lynn K. Nyhart, 225–48. Chicago: University of Chicago Press, 2017.

Latour, Bruno. *An Inquiry into Modes of Existence: An Anthropology of the Moderns*. Translated by Catherine Porter. Cambridge, MA: Harvard University Press, 2013.

———. *Pandora's Hope: Essays on the Reality of Science Studies*. Cambridge, MA: Harvard University Press, 1999.

———. *The Pasteurization of France*. Translated by Alan Sheridan and John Law. Cambridge, MA: Harvard University Press, 1988.

Latour, Bruno, and Peter Weibel. *Making Things Public: Atmospheres of Democracy*. Cambridge, MA: MIT Press, 2005.

Latour, Bruno, and Steve Woolgar. *Laboratory Life: The Construction of Scientific Facts*. Princeton, NJ: Princeton University Press, 1986.

Lau, D. C., and Roger T. Ames, trans. *Yuan Dao: Tracing Dao to Its Source*. New York: Ballantine Books, 1998.

Law, John. "What's Wrong with a One-World World?" *Distinktion: Journal of Social Theory* 16, no. 1 (August 2015): 126–39.

Law, John, and Wen-yuan Lin. "Provincializing STS: Postcoloniality, Symmetry, and Method." *East Asian Science, Technology and Society (EASTS)* 11, no. 2 (2017): 211–27.

Lei, Sean Hsiang-lin. *Neither Donkey nor Horse: Medicine in the Struggle over China's Modernity*. Chicago: University of Chicago Press, 2014.

Leslie, Charles. "The Ambiguities of Medical Revivalism in Modern India." In *Asian Medical Systems: A Comparative Study*, edited by Charles Leslie, 356–67. Berkeley: University of California Press, 1976.

Liao, Yuqun 廖育群. 医者意也：认识中医 *Yizhe Yi ye: Renshi Zhongyi* [Medicine Is Thought: Knowing Chinese Medicine]. Nanning: Guangxi Normal University Press, 2006.

Liu, Lydia He. *Translingual Practice: Literature, National Culture, and Translated Modernity—China, 1900–1937*. Stanford, CA: Stanford University Press, 1995.

Lloyd, Geoffrey, and Nathan Sivin. *The Way and the Word: Science and Medicine in Early China and Greece.* New Haven, CT: Yale University Press, 2002.

Lopez, Donald S. *The Scientific Buddha: His Short and Happy Life.* New Haven, CT: Yale University Press, 2012.

Lu, Guangxin 陆广莘. 中医学之道. *Zhongyixue Zhi Dao* [The Way of Chinese Medicine]. Beijing: People's Health Press, 2001.

Lu, Gwei-Djen, and Joseph Needham. *Celestial Lancets: A History and Rationale of Acupuncture and Moxa.* Cambridge: Cambridge University Press, 1980.

Mao, Zedong. "On Contradiction." In *Selected Works of Mao Tse-Tung,* 85–133. Beijing: Foreign Language Press, 1967.

———. "On Practice." In *Selected Works of Mao Tse-Tung,* 295–309. Beijing: Foreign Language Press, 1967.

———. *Serve the People.* Peking: Foreign Languages Press, 1966.

Mead, Margaret. *Continuities in Cultural Evolution.* New Haven, CT: Yale University Press, 1964.

Mitchell, Timothy. "Can the Mosquito Speak?" In *Rule of Experts: Egypt, Techno-Politics, Modernity,* 19–53. Berkeley: University of California Press, 2002.

Montgomery, Kathryn. *How Doctors Think: Clinical Judgment and the Practice of Medicine.* Oxford: Oxford University Press, 2006.

Montgomery, Sy. *The Soul of an Octopus: A Joyful Exploration into the Wonder of Consciousness.* New York: Atria Books, 2015.

Morris, Ivan I., ed. *Madly Singing in the Mountains: An Appreciation and Anthology of Arthur Waley.* New York: Walker, 1970.

Murthy, Viren. *The Political Philosophy of Zhang Taiyan: The Resistance of Consciousness.* Leiden: Brill, 2011.

Nappi, Carla Suzan. *The Monkey and the Inkpot: Natural History and Its Transformations in Early Modern China.* Cambridge, MA: Harvard University Press, 2009.

Needham, Joseph. *The Grand Titration: Science and Society in East and West.* London: Allen & Unwin, 1969.

————. *Science and Civilisation in China.* 7 vols. Cambridge: Cambridge University Press, 1954–2004.

————. *Science and Civilisation in China.* Vol. 2. Cambridge: Cambridge University Press, 1956.

Niranjana, Tejaswini. *Siting Translation: History, Post-Structuralism, and the Colonial Context.* Berkeley: University of California Press, 1992.

Ou, Ming 欧明, ed. 汉英中医词典 *Han Ying Zhong Yi Ci Dian* [Chinese-English Dictionary of Traditional Chinese Medicine]. Guangzhou: Guangzhou Science and Technology Press, 1986.

Pickering, Andrew. *Constructing Quarks: A Sociological History of Particle Physics.* Chicago: University of Chicago Press, 1984.

————. *The Mangle of Practice: Time, Agency, and Science.* Chicago: University of Chicago Press, 1995.

Porkert, Manfred. *The Theoretical Foundations of Chinese Medicine: Systems of Correspondence.* Cambridge, MA: MIT Press, 1974.

Qin, Bowei 秦伯未. 中医入门 *Zhongyi Rumen* [Introduction to Chinese Medicine]. Beijing: People's Health Press, 1959.

Ren, Yingqiu 任应秋. 通俗中国医学史话 *Tongsu Zhongguo Yixue Shihua* [On China's Medical History]. Chongqing: Chongqing People's Press, 1957.

Rheinberger, Hans-Jörg. *An Epistemology of the Concrete: Twentieth-Century Histories of Life.* Durham, NC: Duke University Press, 2010.

Ricoeur, Paul. *Freud and Philosophy: An Essay on Interpretation.* New Haven, CT: Yale University Press, 1970.

Sapir, Edward. "The Unconscious Patterning of Behavior in Society." In *Language, Culture, and Society: A Book of Readings,* edited by Ben G. Blount, 29–42. Prospect Heights, IL: Waveland Press, 1995.

Saunders, Barry F. *CT Suite: The Work of Diagnosis in the Age of Noninvasive Cutting.* Durham, NC: Duke University Press, 2008.

Scheid, Volker. *Chinese Medicine in Contemporary China: Plurality and Synthesis.* Durham, NC: Duke University Press, 2002.

————. *Currents of Tradition in Chinese Medicine, 1626–2006.* Seattle: Eastland Press, 2007.

Scheid, Volker, and Curie Virág. "Introduction to History of Science Special Section on *Tong*." *History of Science* 56, no. 2 (June 2018): 123–30.

Schipper, Kristofer Marinus. *The Taoist Body*. Berkeley: University of California Press, 1993.

Scorzon, Cinzia. "Tong 通 in Clinical Acupuncture Practice." *Translating Vitalities* (blog), October 2018, https://translatingvitalities.com/what/.

Sidel, Victor W., and Ruth Sidel. *Serve the People: Observations on Medicine in the People's Republic of China.* New York: Josiah Macy, Jr., Foundation, 1973.

Sigerist, Henry E. *Medicine and Human Welfare*. New Haven, CT: Yale University Press, 1941.

Sivin, Nathan. *Traditional Medicine in Contemporary China: A Partial Translation of Revised Outline of Chinese Medicine (1972): With an Introductory Study on Change in Present Day and Early Medicine.* Ann Arbor: Center for Chinese Studies, University of Michigan, 1987.

Smith, Barbara Herrnstein. *Contingencies of Value: Alternative Perspectives for Critical Theory.* Cambridge, MA: Harvard University Press, 1988.

———. *Natural Reflections: Human Cognition at the Nexus of Science and Religion.* New Haven, CT: Yale University Press, 2009.

———. *Practicing Relativism in the Anthropocene: On Science, Belief, and the Humanities.* Ann Arbor, MI: Open Humanities Press, 2018.

———. "Religion, Science, and the Humanities: An Interview." In *Practicing Relativism in the Anthropocene: On Science, Belief, and the Humanities,* 32–39. Ann Arbor, MI: Open Humanities Press, 2018.

Smith, Paul. *Discerning the Subject.* Minneapolis: University of Minnesota Press, 1988.

Stanley-Baker, Michael. "Health and Philosophy in Pre- and Early Imperial China." In *Health and Philosophy,* edited by Peter Adamson, 7–42. Oxford: Oxford University Press, forthcoming.

Taylor, Kim. *Chinese Medicine in Early Communist China, 1945–63: A Medicine of Revolution.* London: RoutledgeCurzon, 2005.

Thomas, William Isaac, and Dorothy Swaine Thomas. *The Child in America: Behavior Problems and Programs.* New York: Alfred A. Knopf, 1928.

Van Fraassen, Bas C. *The Empirical Stance*. New Haven, CT: Yale University Press, 2002.

Verran, Helen. "On Assemblage: Indigenous Knowledge and Digital Media (2003–2006) and HMS Investigator (1800–1805)." In *Assembling Culture*, edited by Tony Bennet and Chris Healey, 163–76. London: Routledge, 2011.

Wang, Jun. "A Life History of Ren Yingqiu: Historical Problems, Mythology, Continuity and Difference in Chinese Medical Modernity." PhD diss., University of North Carolina at Chapel Hill, 2003.

Wiseman, Nigel, and Ye Feng. *A Practical Dictionary of Chinese Medicine*. Brookline, MA: Paradigm Publications, 1998.

Wong, Chimin, and Lien-teh Wu. *History of Chinese Medicine: Being a Chronicle of Medical Happenings in China from Ancient Times to the Present Period*. Tientsin: Tientsin Press, 1932.

Xie, Guan 谢观. 中国医学源流论 *Zhongguo Yixue Yuanliulun* [Sources and Currents of Chinese Medicine]. Fuzhou: Fujian Science and Technology Press.

Yin, Huihe 印会河, ed. 中医基础理论 *Zhongyi Jichu Lilun* [Basic Theory of Chinese Medicine]. Shanghai: Shanghai Science and Technology Press, 1982.

Young, Allan. "The Discourse on Stress and the Reproduction of Conventional Knowledge." *Social Science and Medicine (Part B. Medical Anthropology)* 14, no. 3 (August 1980): 133–46.

Zhan, Mei. *Other-Worldly: Making Chinese Medicine through Transnational Frames*. Durham, NC: Duke University Press, 2009.

Zhang, Dong 张东. 元气 神机：先秦中医之道 *Yuanqi Shenji: Xianqin Zhongyi zhi Dao* [Original Qi: Vital Machine]. Xi'an: World Book Publishers, 2016.

Zhang, Qicheng 张其成. 中医哲学基础 *Zhongyi Zhexue Jichu* [Philosophical Foundations of Chinese Medicine]. Beijing: Chinese Medicine Press of China, 2004.

Zhang, Yanhua. *Transforming Emotions with Chinese Medicine: An Ethnographic Account from Contemporary China*. Albany: State University of New York Press, 2007.

Zhuang, Zhou 庄周. 庄子全译 *Zhuangzi Quanyi* [The Complete Zhuangzi with Commentary]. Commentator Gengguang Zhang 张耿光. Guiyang: Guizhou People's Press, 1991.

Index

Boxes, figures, notes, and tables are denoted by *b, f, n,* and *t* following the page number.

four examinations, 59–65, 60*b*, 70,
  71, 86–87, 146*n*16
Fox, Renée, 150*n*20

Galison, Peter, 143*n*38
Garon, Colin, 89, 143*n*41
Geaney, Jane, 146*n*14
Geertz, Clifford, 3
Guangzhou College of Traditional
  Chinese Medicine, 1–2

He Yiren, 88
headaches, 103–4
Heidegger, Martin, 20, 143*n*39,
  144*n*53
herbalists and herbalism, 31, 58, 79,
  85, 87, 88–90*b*, 91, 93–94, 120,
  122, 146*n*12. *See also* drugs and drug
  formulas; prescriptions
Huainanzi, 144*n*50
Huang Jitang, 3–4
Huang Lao School, 130, 131
Huang Moya, 124
Huangdi Neijing (*Inner Canon of the
  Yellow Emperor*), 80, 122–33, 136,
  141n26
hypochondria, 148–49*n*8

Indian traditional medicine, 142*n*28
infratranslation, 11
Inner Canon of the Yellow Emperor.
  See *Huangdi Neijing*
Introduction to Chinese Medicine
  (*Zhongyi Rumen*), 64. *See also* Qin
  Bowei

James, William, 1, 14, 15, 19, 33–34,
  45, 47, 61, 146*n*17

Jaspers, Karl, 121, 124
Jensen, Casper Bruun, 137*n*6,
  143*n*38
Jullien, François, 144*n*53, 152*n*10,
  153*n*17

kanbing (looking at illness), 84,
  86–88, 91
Kaptchuk, Ted, 55, 115, 116, 140*n*8,
  145*n*6, 151*nn*2–3
Kuriyama, Shigehisa, 144*n*51

Lai Lili, 94, 121
Laozi, 129, 130, 132
Latour, Bruno, 21, 144*n*53
Lau, D. C., 147*n*31
Law, John, 5, 16, 144*n*53
Lenin: *What Is to Be Done?
  Burning Questions of Our Time*,
  151*n*7
li fa fang yao (patterns, disciplines,
  formulas, medicines), 52, 53–56*b*,
  53*f*, 56–59, 63, 64, 147*n*21
Li Shizhen, 93, 150*n*15
Liao Yuqun, 66, 75–76, 93–95,
  144*n*1, 146*n*14, 149*n*13
life gate (*mingmen*), 9–10, 17,
  147*n*30
Lin, Wen-yuan, 144*n*53
Lloyd, Geoffrey, 114, 115
Lopez, Donald, 3
Lu Guangxin, 34–37, 44–45, 66, 94,
  107–10
Lu Gwei-Djen, 5–8, 9–12*b*,
  138–39*n*15, 138*n*10

Mao Zedong, 28, 82, 109, 117
Mead, Margaret, 3